CONTENTS

Introduction   iii

1. What Is Fatty Liver?   1
2. How Serious Can A Fatty Liver Be?   14
3. Understanding Fatty Liver Disease   20
4. Fatty Liver Diagnosis And Treatment   32
5. Fatty Liver Diet Foods   42
6. Things you Should Know to Reduce Fat in Your Liver   51
7. How To Eliminate A Fatty Liver Problem   60
8. Weight Loss For Fatty Liver Disease   79
9. How To Successfully Combat A Fatty Liver   105
10. Fatty Liver Disease is a Ticking Time Bomb: Get Yourself Examined Today   114

Conclusion   137

INTRODUCTION

Fatty liver is the build-up of fats within the liver cells to the point that more than 5-10% of the liver is fat. Fatty liver is a condition in which fat accumulates in the liver cells. However, the simple fatty liver does not damage the liver. Fat accumulation in the liver can be caused by weight gain or diabetes mellitus. Fatty liver can occur with a lean diet and ailments such as tuberculosis and intestinal bypass surgery for obesity. It can also occur while certain drugs like corticosteroids. The condition is also caused by heavy alcohol use. A patient is diagnosed as having a fatty liver when fat makes up at least 10% of the liver.

Fatty food does not cause a fatty liver. It is a common condition that is seen in people who are overweight or have diabetes. Explanations for a fatty liver include the transfer of fat from other parts of the body or a spurt in the extraction of fat presented to the liver from the intestine. Another argument is that the fat accumulates because the liver cannot change it into a form that can be removed.

INTRODUCTION

Fatty liver is diagnosed by eliminating the chances of chronic liver disease, particularly from alcohol abuse. Images of the liver obtained through an ultrasound test, a CT scan, or a magnetic resonance imaging (MRI) scan can diagnose a fatty liver. In an ultrasound test, a fatty liver produces a bright image in a ripple pattern. A CT scan will show a picture in which the liver will appear less dense than normal.

The treatment of fatty liver is linked with the cause. A simple fatty liver does not need treatment because it does not damage the liver cells. Overweight patients with fatty liver will have to reduce their weight. Control of diabetes also decreases the fat content in the liver.

Another condition that causes fat deposit in the liver is nonalcoholic steatohepatitis (NASH). But, unlike a simple fatty liver, it causes damage to the liver cells. It is not linked to other causes of chronic liver disease, like hepatitis B and C viruses, autoimmune disorders, alcohol, drug toxicity, copper accumulation (Wilson's Disease), or iron (hemochromatosis).

The first question that comes to mind when being diagnosed with fatty liver disease is this: is there a treatment for this disease? There are ways to reverse the disease and the symptoms you have. A healthy lifestyle plays a vital role in sickness; however, it can reverse fatty liver disease.

What is fatty liver disease? It is also known as hepatic steatosis, in which the liver malfunctions due to the excess amounts of fat build-up in the liver. Fat will build up in the liver, carried by the bloodstream to various parts of the body, especially in places where we do not want it the most. Without making any changes in diet and exercise, the liver continues to accumulate fat deposits, which can lead to other various health problems, such as obesity and diabetes mellitus type II.

INTRODUCTION

So, how do we change our diet to get rid of this unwanted liver illness?

Simple. We need to decrease the intake of high-fat foods instead of consuming low-fat, non-fat foods. Nowadays, we are given the luxury to choose foods with low-fat content, such as milk and yogurt, to name a few examples. Initially, our taste palates are used to high fat-containing foods, but starting slowly with simple things, you will no longer desire to intake high-fat foods. Other ways to have a healthy diet are consuming high fiber foods, such as fruits and vegetables. This can allow you to feel full longer and provide the body with essential vitamins and minerals. Taking the diet seriously can reverse fatty liver disease, and you will immediately notice differences: waistline decreasing, feeling more energized.

Diet and exercise go hand in hand. It is not enough with eating right to reverse this fatty disease process; it is also important to incorporate exercise. Going for walks, hitting the gym with a couple of friends, finding a trainer to introduce healthy workout habits are just some of the few ways to start. By eating well and exercising well, our bodies have the essential nutrients to keep our energy levels higher, and improve our blood circulation, respectively.

Who Gets Fatty Liver Disease?

About one in 10 Americans are affected by this condition – it's the most common reason for abnormal liver test results. An excessive alcohol intake often causes fatty liver disease. Still, it is increasingly being found in people who do not drink to excess but are overweight or obese or have diabetes. Non-alcoholic fatty liver disease (NAFLD) affects one in 3 adults and is the most common cause of chronic liver disease. It's even being diagnosed in American teenagers.

INTRODUCTION

Read on to understand the fatty liver symptoms and how to reverse your fatty liver naturally.

WHAT IS FATTY LIVER?

Fatty liver refers to a group of conditions in which there is an excessive accumulation of fat in the liver. Normally, various types of fat, including triglycerides and cholesterol, are metabolized in this organ. However, in this condition, an abnormal amount of fat accumulates in the cells of this organ, despite the absence of alcohol consumption. In fact, in some patients, this illness is associated with inflammation and scarring of the liver, eventually leading to cirrhosis, a condition in which liver cells are mostly replaced by scar tissue. This illness is a prevalent condition affecting up to 20% of the adult population. Obesity is the most common cause of this condition. Up to 75% of obese individuals are found to have this condition.

The majority of patients with this condition do not have any symptoms. Fatty liver is most often diagnosed on a routine blood test in an otherwise asymptomatic individual. There is a mild degree of elevation of liver enzymes called ALT and AST in patients with fatty liver. The diagnosis of the fatty liver requires imaging studies of the liver such as ultrasound. To confirm the diagnosis of fatty liver, common causes known to elevate the liver enzymes, including certain medications, viral hepatitis, autoimmune liver disease, and inherited liver disease, need to be excluded. The most reliable means of diagnosing fatty liver is by performing a liver biopsy, although rarely necessary to establish the diagnosis of fatty liver.

Most patients with this clinical condition have little or no problem, but up to 25% of patients may develop chronic scarring of the liver due to chronic inflammation in this organ. This may lead to a complication known as cirrhosis, where most liver cells are replaced by scar tissue. In cirrhosis, the liver cannot function properly due to an insufficient number of functioning cells in this organ. Patients with cirrhosis often develop bleeding, fluid in the abdomen called ascites, yellowing of the skin or jaundice, and even confusion and altered level of consciousness. These patients may eventually require transplantation of the liver. Also, there appears to be a significant risk of developing the cancer of the liver, called hepatocellular carcinoma.

The treatment of fatty liver involves weight reduction, dietary modification, increased physical activity, and excessive alcohol and unnecessary medication. It is also important to control diabetes and cholesterol in patients who are affected by these conditions.

Fatty liver disease, or FLD, is the condition that marks an excessive accumulation of fat within the cells of the liver. This condition is not considered normal for any individual, but it is not likely to permanently damage nature.

However, individuals who experience an accumulation of fat in this organ may experience other health complications that could negatively impact their overall health. One of the main health concerns that individuals with fatty liver may experience is inflammation of the liver.

Once this occurs, it could result in the onset of scarring of the liver. This is referred to as cirrhosis. This is considered to be one of the most serious of all liver-related medical conditions.

Types of Fatty Liver

There are two main types of fatty liver disease: nonalcoholic and alcoholic.

Nonalcoholic fatty liver disease (NAFLD) includes simple nonalcoholic fatty liver, nonalcoholic steatohepatitis (NASH), and acute fatty liver of pregnancy (AFLP). Alcoholic fatty liver disease (AFLD) includes simple AFLD and alcoholic steatohepatitis (ASH).

- *Nonalcoholic fatty liver disease (NAFLD).*

Nonalcoholic fatty liver disease (NAFLD) occurs when fat builds up in the liver of people who don't drink a lot of alcohol. If you have excess fat in your liver and no history of heavy alcohol use, your doctor may diagnose you with NAFLD.

If there's no inflammation or other complications and the build-up of fat, the condition is known as a simple nonalcoholic fatty liver.

- *Nonalcoholic steatohepatitis (NASH).*

Nonalcoholic steatohepatitis (NASH) is a type of NAFLD. It occurs when a build-up of excess fat in the liver is accompanied by liver inflammation.

If you have excess fat in your liver, your liver is inflamed, and you have no history of heavy alcohol use, your doctor may diagnose you with NASH. When left untreated, NASH can cause scarring of your liver. In severe cases, this can lead to cirrhosis and liver failure.

- *Acute fatty liver of pregnancy (AFLP).*

Acute fatty liver of pregnancy (AFLP) is a rare but severe complication of pregnancy. The exact cause is unknown.

When AFLP develops, it usually appears in the third trimester of pregnancy. If left untreated, it poses serious health risks to the mother and growing baby.

If you're diagnosed with AFLP, your doctor will want to deliver your baby as soon as possible. You might need to receive follow-up care for several days after you give birth. Your liver health will likely return to normal within a few weeks of giving birth.

- *Alcoholic fatty liver disease (ALFD).*

Drinking a lot of alcohol damages the liver. When it's damaged, the liver can't break down fat properly. This can cause fat to build up, which is known as alcoholic fatty liver. Alcoholic fatty liver disease (ALFD) is the earliest stage of alcohol-related liver disease.

If there's no inflammation or other complications and the build-up of fat, the condition is known as simple alcoholic fatty liver.

- *Alcoholic steatohepatitis (ASH).*

Alcoholic steatohepatitis (ASH) is a type of AFLD. It happens when a build-up of excess fat in the liver is accompanied by liver inflammation. This is also known as alcoholic hepatitis.

If you have excess fat in your liver, your liver is inflamed, and you drink a lot of alcohol, your doctor may diagnose you with ASH.

If it's not treated properly, ASH can cause scarring of your liver. Severe liver scarring is known as cirrhosis. It can lead to liver failure.

To treat alcoholic fatty liver, it's important to avoid alcohol. If you have alcoholism or alcohol use disorder, your doctor may recommend counseling or other treatments.

Causes of Fatty Liver

Fatty liver is the accumulation of fat in liver cells; possible explanations of fatty liver include the transfer of fat from other parts of the body or an increase in the extraction of fat presented to the liver from the intestine. Other explanations are that the liver reduces the rate it breaks down and removes fat; eating fatty foods does not by itself produce a fatty liver.

Did you know that 33% of the American population suffers from fatty liver and doesn't know about it? Fatty liver, or steatosis, is the accumulation of fat inside liver cells. This fat takes up precious resources and leads to mild liver failure that can grow into cirrhosis and full-blown liver failure. The causes of steatosis are multiple, but, fortunately, this is a reversible disorder.

The main cause of fatty liver today is obesity. Eating too much fat or sugar stresses the liver, which must process it. It develops steatosis, and its function of burning fat is compromised, reducing metabolism and making weight loss difficult.

Another major culprit is alcohol. Alcohol puts too much stress on the liver's detoxifying function, killing cells that are replaced by non-functional fibrotic tissue (cirrhosis). Drugs (even doctor prescribed and homeopathic remedies) act in the same way, though they are not as aggressive as alcohol. Unless you are overdosing, your liver can regenerate faster than these drugs damage it.

Even if you are not obese and don't take drugs or alcohol, you can still have steatosis. This happens when your diet is not healthy - if you eat too much meat and few vegetables or fruit, your liver will be damaged, even if your silhouette doesn't show it.

Many are under the misconception that a fatty liver is based on how much fat-filled foods a person consumes. In all actuality, medical professionals are still struggling with identifying one particular cause of this condition. It has been established that the liver plays a significant role in the process of metabolism that involves breaking down fats in the body.

It is believed that some error is experienced in this process, and much of the fat is retained in this organ. Individuals that are overweight or are considered to be obese often experience this condition. If an individual has a high level of triglycerides in the body, they are likely to suffer from a fatty liver.

Individuals that have certain health complications such as diabetes and tuberculosis may experience this liver problem. It is also common for those that take certain medications and drink alcohol heavily to develop this problem.

What Causes Fatty Liver in Slim People?

There are 2 types of sugar monomers, glucose and fructose (other sugars like lactose, sucrose are disaccharides made of glucose and fructose).

When you eat glucose, it's absorbed into your bloodstream and goes to power your muscles, brain, etc. If there's too much, your pancreas produces extra insulin to tell your body to store that glucose as fat (subcutaneous mostly).

When you eat fructose, some of it is converted to glucose before absorption, and the rest goes essentially directly to your liver. In the liver, it is changed into either 1) glycogen or 2) triglycerides (fatty acids).

If your liver is depleted of glycogen (after a hard endurance workout), most fructose will replenish the glycogen, so it doesn't create much of a problem.

If, on the other hand, you already have enough glycogen, or you eat a lot of fructose in a rapidly absorbable form (like HFCS or agave nectar), then it will mostly be converted to triglycerides.

Some of those triglycerides will be released into your bloodstream, either to be stored as fat (depending on how much insulin has been circulating) or to be burned for fuel (depending on how much work your body and brain are doing, assuming that there isn't much insulin floating around).

The rest, of course, will be stored right there in the liver in case your body ever needs them. If you do not exercise enough to demand those triglycerides from your liver (and to be fair, they are released from the liver, usually before they are released from your stored fat cells), then the fat builds up over time and gets fatty liver.

So, when you see someone slim with fatty liver (non-alcoholic), it usually means that they have been getting too much fructose and have not been doing the type of exercise needed to burn off the liver glycogen and/or liver triglycerides (usually endurance exercise, but Interval Training and weight training can also contribute, depending on the duration and format of the total workout).

All that said, it seems to me that it's pretty hard to get the fatty liver disease from non-liquefied sources. Yes, fruits have fructose, and so do many other things. But if consumed in the whole form, the absorption is slower, and the bulkiness of the food usually limits the total dose. In general, the problem is with liquid sugars, especially high-fructose sugars. Although some have suggested that fructose+glucose may even be worse for your health, it probably would not lead to the combo of slimness+NAFLD.

Fatty Livers: A Silent Cause of Premature Death

The liver is the largest and most under-rated organ in the human body. It's often described as the body's chemical factory since it's responsible for at least five hundred vital human functions. These include cleansing the blood, detoxifying poisons, fighting infections, manufacturing proteins, and processing digested foods. The importance of these life-preserving tasks was recognized by our ancestors, who called the liver 'the seat of life.' That's how it gained its name, which comes from the Anglo-Saxon word libban, meaning 'to live.'

Owing to its importance, the liver is provided with amazing powers of regeneration. If 90 percent of a dog's liver is excised, it will regain its full size within six to eight weeks. The Greeks recognized this remarkable resilience in their legend of Prometheus, the mortal who stole fire from the gods and brought it back to earth. He was punished by Zeus, who had him tied to a rock, where a giant eagle ate his liver every day, only to have it re-grow during the hours of darkness. In recent years, something has happened to impair these astonishing powers of regeneration. Statistics show that liver disease is now the fifth major cause of death in the United States. Experts warn that unless preventive measures are taken in the next ten to twenty years, it could well overtake coronary disease and stroke as England's major cause of death.

What's more alarming, many of these fatalities will arise when people are relatively young, for the average age of death from liver disease is 59, compared with 82 for someone who dies of a stroke. But the news is not all bad, for it's estimated that 95 percent of these deaths are preventable. They were associated with excessive alcohol consumption, virus infections, and toxic reaction to drugs like paracetamol. Now they're increasingly linked with obesity.

One of the liver's key functions is to process, manufacture and regulate the supply of triglycerides, which are the body's major fat sources. This is an automated function, and in a state of health, there should be little or no residual fat accumulating in the liver. But this can change if the bloodstream is overloaded with fat. The Egyptians discovered this in 2500BC, who found that they could enlarge the livers of geese by restricting their activities and force-feeding them at regular intervals. Their livers became swollen with fat, which made a delightful paté known as foie gras or 'fat liver.' We're doing the same thing; the only difference is that the geese were killed to obtain their livers, whereas we're being slain by our diseased livers, which have no use as foods and are too damaged to be used for liver transplants.

Today, as a direct effect of the obesity plague, it's reckoned that one in five British adults is now suffering from fatty liver disease, unconnected with virus infections or heavy drinking. This disorder, known medically as steatosis, is believed to affect 90 percent of morbidly obese patients, in whom it may remain symptomless for many years. During this time, it causes inflammation in the tissues surrounding the fat-filled cells, which, if prolonged, can give rise to cirrhosis and premature death unless its victims are given the benefit of a liver transplant. This operation has practically doubled in recent years in the US. If forecasts prove correct, half a million obese children in the US could risk developing fatty liver disease. This means that many will die in their 50s and 60s unless they're encouraged to shed their excess pounds. For safety's sake, Mother Nature has provided us with two eyes and two kidneys. But we're born with only one liver, which has to work night and day to preserve our vitality and health. So, if you want to lead a long and vigorous life, take steps to protect your liver.

Symptoms of Fatty Liver

Learning to recognize the symptoms of a fatty liver is important as this is typically the way to diagnose alcoholic or non-alcoholic liver disease. Fat that shows up on much of the body is tough to ignore. You cannot shut your eyes to belly and leg fat, but liver fat is completely different. You do not feel or see your liver, so liver fat is often not noticed. All livers do contain some fat, but once the fat reaches more than 10 percent, there is often a problem with the liver.

While the fatty liver can result in serious health consequences, it is not often that a patient experiences actual symptoms. Nearly all cases of this liver problem are identified through an examination or a medical evaluation that is working to determine if the patient is experiencing another issue.

There are blood tests that can determine the amount of liver-based enzymes in the blood. In other instances, an electronic imaging test such as a CAT Scan, MRI, or ultrasound may identify the fact that the liver is swollen or inflamed. If a doctor suspects that the liver may contain a lot of fat, they can immediately diagnose it.

However, some medical professionals will elect to perform a biopsy to confirm a diagnosis. If you have been informed that you suffer from fatty liver or fatty liver disease, it is important to work directly with your doctor on a treatment plan. By doing so, you may be able to reverse the damage that has been done to this vital organ.

Mild cases of fatty liver generally do not have noticeable symptoms. However, numerous health conditions may alert you that you are at risk or already have fatty liver disease. **These include:**

- Overweight or obesity
- Chronic lack of energy
- Tiredness and fatigue
- High blood sugar
- Insulin Resistance or Diabetes
- Metabolic Syndrome
- Chronic congestion
- Skin rashes and breakouts
- Possibly, allergies and other sensitivities
- Bruising
- Hypertension
- Gall stones or gall bladder disease
- Chronic yeast or urinary infections
- Drinking excessive amounts of alcohol
- Intense cravings for sugar or carbs

Women with fatty liver also struggle with:

- Menstrual Irregularities
- Low Energy and Depression
- Hormone Imbalances
- Ovarian Cysts (PCOS)

Fatty liver is often diagnosed when treated for another condition and is usually found on a routine blood test.

In its early stages, you may notice rashes and breakouts on your skin--well, before you know your liver is being affected. If fatty liver is not treated in its early stages, your liver can become swollen and inflamed.

To quickly summarize the cause: Your liver is responsible for metabolizing (breaking down) and storing fats, sugars, and carbohydrates from the foods you eat. During metabolism, excess fats, sugars or carbs build up in your liver cells and are stored in liver tissues as fatty deposits. Your liver is also responsible for cleansing toxins, which are a normal by-product of the metabolic process. When an excessive amount of fatty buildup overwhelms your liver cells and tissues, it causes inflammation. Over time, this chronic inflammation causes swelling and liver enlargement.

When your liver is struggling to metabolize fats and cleanse toxins and is overwhelmed with an accumulation of fatty deposits, it becomes swollen and inflamed.

This is when you start noticing the symptoms: Fatigue, nausea, burning sensation in your stomach, and abdominal or back pain. This is a sign that a harmful condition is at work in your body!

If left untreated, the inflammation and swelling can damage your liver cells and lead to a more serious diagnosis of Steatohepatitis (NASH).

In severe cases, the inflammation and swelling cause liver cells to burst. This cellular injury leads to scarring of the liver (cirrhosis) and irreversible liver damage.

The simple truth is... If you feel the symptoms of fatty liver or have already been diagnosed, that means your liver is already swollen, inflamed, and under extreme stress.

Fatty liver disease is, as noted, hard to recognize as symptoms often take decades to present themselves. If you experience symptoms of a fatty liver, make an appointment with your doctor for a blood test or other diagnosis method. This diagnosis allows the doctor to start the appropriate treatment regimen, preventing further disease and destruction.

Fatty Liver Risk Factors

Drinking high amounts of alcohol puts you at increased risk of developing fatty liver. **You may also be at heightened risk if you:**

- are obese
- have insulin resistance
- have type 2 diabetes
- have polycystic ovary syndrome
- are pregnant
- have a history of certain infections, such as hepatitis C
- take certain medications, such as methotrexate (Trexall), tamoxifen (Nolvadex), amiodarone (Pacerone), and valproic acid (Depakote)
- have high cholesterol levels
- have high triglyceride levels
- have high blood sugar levels
- have metabolic syndrome

Risk factors for alcoholic liver disease

- Not surprisingly, the risk factor for this type of fatty liver disease is drinking too much alcohol.

If you have a family history of fatty liver disease, you're more likely to develop it yourself.

HOW SERIOUS CAN A FATTY LIVER BE?

In most cases, the fatty liver disease doesn't cause any serious problems or prevent your liver from functioning normally. But for 7% to 30% of people with the condition, the fatty liver disease gets worse over time. **It progresses through three stages:**

- Your liver becomes inflamed (swollen), which damages its tissue. This stage is called steatohepatitis.
- Scar tissue forms where your liver is damaged. This process is called fibrosis.
- Extensive scar tissue replaces healthy tissue. At this point, you have cirrhosis of the liver.

CIRRHOSIS OF THE LIVER

. . .

CIRRHOSIS OF THE LIVER IS A RESULT OF SEVERE DAMAGE TO THE LIVER. The hard scar tissue that replaces healthy liver tissue slows down the liver's functioning. Eventually, it can block liver function entirely. Cirrhosis can lead to liver failure and liver cancer.

Facts You May Find Surprising About Liver Disease

THE SEVERITY OF THE LIVER DISEASE CAN RANGE DRAMATICALLY FROM mild and manageable to debilitating and eventually even fatal. If the liver disease can be treated early enough and if the treatment is followed, most liver disease can be managed. The liver is a very durable organ, but it is asked to do so much we want it to work as efficiently as possible. **Here are a few common myths that could prevent efforts to detect liver disease if not fully understood:**

1. **Disease of the liver can be cured with a liver transplant.** Since this is considered the last resort to keep a person alive when the liver is destroyed, the recipient might feel that they're out of the woods with a transplant. There are still things that can go wrong. The body may reject a new liver or the recipient that still falls prey to the same thing that caused the first liver to fail.

1. **Fatty liver disease is not a big problem.** Because so many people now are afflicted with fatty liver and seem to be doing okay, it might not seem to be such a big deal. Non-alcoholic fatty liver disease is carried by between a quarter and a third of all Americans today. In its earliest

HEALTH AND WELLNESS LIFE

stages, the person might not even know they have the disease, but it can be the precursor of more serious issues such as cirrhosis of the liver. This can lead to liver cancer and liver failure. It should be looked at as an issue that should be addressed as soon as possible.

1. **Disease of the liver is caused by alcoholism.** Excessive alcohol can cause liver damage, but it is only one cause of over 100 forms of liver disease. Alcoholic hepatitis is often found in alcoholics but can also be found in people who are not. It is very hard to predict how the liver is going to react to alcohol, and if alcohol is the problem, the situation is often reversed for those who stop drinking.

1. **Hepatitis C only comes from drug addiction.** One of the foremost causes of liver disease is hepatitis C, and it can indeed be acquired from the sharing of intravenous needles. But adults who were exposed to hepatitis C before it was started to be screened in 1992 could have been exposed without ever having come into contact with contaminated needles.

1. **Diseases of the liver are only an adult issue.** Liver issues typically occur in adults who frankly don't do a good job taking care of their liver over a long time. But there are approximately 15,000 children who are hospitalized every year with liver disorders. The major causes are hepatitis A,

B, and C viruses, blockages in bile flow, and genetic issues. Obese children are also at a high risk of getting fatty liver disease.

HAVING A BETTER AWARENESS OF LIVER PROBLEMS WILL HELP FOR AN early diagnosis, and that is the best defense for a diseased liver that can eventually be out of control. The best cure for liver damage is to manage the causes before the inflammation severely damages the liver's cells.

How To Know If You Can Live A Long Life With A Fatty Liver

FATTY LIVER IS A COMMON AFFLICTION FOR OVERWEIGHT/CONSUME excessive alcohol/have an unhealthy diet with a surfeit of saturated fat/subsist on packaged junk food, prone to a sedentary lifestyle with little exercise.

MANY PEOPLE ARE PROBABLY NOT EVEN AWARE THEY HAVE A FATTY liver unless a USG is done.

MILD FATTY LIVER IS REVERSIBLE WITH FEW LIFESTYLE CHANGES/GIVING up on excessive alcohol consumption; medication also helps. Neglecting it can, however, be dangerous. Fatty liver, beyond a stage, can result in acute liver disease, which is life-threatening.

. . .

Is Fatty Liver Curable?

In many cases, it's possible to reverse fatty liver through lifestyle changes. These changes may help prevent liver damage and scarring.

The condition can cause inflammation, damage to your liver, and potentially irreversible scarring if it's not treated. Severe liver scarring is known as cirrhosis.

If you develop cirrhosis, it increases your risk of liver cancer and liver failure. These complications can be fatal. For the best outcome, it's important to follow your doctor's recommended treatment plan and practice an overall healthy lifestyle.

Fatty Liver - Am I a Victim?

There are millions of people worldwide in treatment for fatty liver, and many others suffer from it but are not aware of that. Some medical experts are calling it the "new epidemic in America."

Fatty liver occurs when there is an abnormal accumulation of fat deposits in your liver cells.

Most people ignore the early signs or take them lightly and, for this reason, fail to diagnose them in time. When the person experiences chronic stomach pain, fatigue, or nausea and seeks treatment, only then does he/she realize they were suffering from fatty liver.

IN MOST CASES, FATTY LIVER DISEASE IS A MILD CONDITION THAT IS easy to treat. However, if left untreated, this condition causes inflammation of the liver. This is usually when a person starts to notice the symptoms. Chronic inflammation and damage to the cells can lead to irreversible damage to your liver. In severe cases, the cells may even burst.

IN MEDICAL TERMINOLOGY, THIS DISEASE IS CALLED STEATOSIS. Steatosis comes in two forms: Non-Alcoholic Fatty Liver disease (NAFLD) and Alcoholic Steatosis. NAFLD occurs in those who suffer from obesity, diabetes, metabolic syndrome, or ovarian cysts but seldom or never drink alcohol. Alcoholic Steatosis is a result of the over-consumption of alcohol.

STEATOSIS IS THE MOST REVERSIBLE FORM OF LIVER DISEASE. HOWEVER, if not treated in time, it can progress to cirrhosis (scarring of the liver), which cannot be reversed. Cirrhosis is a serious condition that can result in jaundice, fluid retention, gallstones, intestinal bleeding, and in many cases, even death.

UNDERSTANDING FATTY LIVER DISEASE

AN ESTIMATED 100 million Americans have some form of non-alcoholic fatty liver disease (NAFLD). Considered uncommon 30 years ago, the prevalence of NAFLD has increased in parallel with the rising obesity rate. NAFLD can be reversed with weight loss, but few are available to reduce or stop fibrosis progression, leading to liver failure or cancer.

Non-alcoholic fatty liver disease (as it's technically known) results from an abundance of fat stored in the liver. Especially in its early stages, it may have no symptoms. However, as fat levels in the liver increase, the disease can become more aggressive, causing symptoms like abdominal swelling and pain, red palms, and yellowed eyes and skin due to jaundice.

We don't know what, exactly, triggers the condition, but it's often found in individuals who are overweight or obese or who have high levels of cholesterol, triglycerides, or blood sugar. Older people, diabetics, and those with body fat concentrated in the belly are at the highest risk.

As the disease progresses, its main complication is liver scarring. This can lead to a host of problems, from abdominal fluid build-up and esophageal swelling too, in the most serious cases, cirrhosis, liver cancer, and end-stage liver failure.

Although fatty liver disease is prevalent — the Centers for Disease Control estimates it affects up to a quarter of the population — its lack of symptoms in most cases means it often goes undiagnosed. Typically, doctors find it when tests done for other reasons point to liver problems. A diagnosis is then made through blood tests, procedures, and, sometimes, a liver biopsy.

Doctors usually prescribe weight loss, as there are no drugs approved to treat the condition. For the most severe cases, a liver transplant may be an option.

Understanding NAFLD in Non-Obese Individuals

The pathophysiology and risk factors for the development of NAFLD in non-obese persons are not fully understood. They seem to be closely associated with insulin resistance, elevated levels of triglycerides, small-density low-density lipoprotein, low levels of high-density lipoprotein cholesterol, and alterations in body composition, with some patients who may have a predisposition to genetic polymorphisms. Individuals with NAFLD who do not have the typical risk factors may also develop non-alcoholic steatohepatitis (NASH) and more advanced liver disease progression.

In lean individuals, a lifestyle change for disease management has limited potential. A study discusses the clinical, histological, and genetic features and risk factors for non-obese NAFLD. It highlights areas for future research, including biological mechanisms that may identify novel targets for intervention in this population. This cohort represents one phenotype of interest currently undergoing whole-exome sequencing and analysis as part of Columbia's precision medicine initiative.

Common Questions About Fatty Liver

The liver is one of the most complex organs in the human body. The job description of this organ includes an important role in metabolizing and detoxification. Many individuals suffer from a condition called a fatty liver disease or (FDL). Like any disease to the liver, it's important to catch this before it gets out of hand.

One-third of all Americans suffer from fatty liver. But what is this disease? Is it serious? And is it treatable?

- *What is fatty liver disease?*

Fatty liver disease, known as steatosis, is the accumulation of fat inside the liver cell. That fat comes from your bloodstream and is taken up by the liver, responsible for converting it to sugar or sending it toward fat cells. However, if the liver can't handle all the fat it gets (whether because you eat too much or because it is already overloaded with other tasks), it piles up. It takes up resources, further reducing the liver's ability to destroy fat.

- *Is fatty liver a serious condition?*

In a word, yes. Steatosis causes a series of mild symptoms, like bad breath, circles under the eyes, and headaches. Because the liver is responsible for burning fat, and ill liver causes obesity (and hard to get rid of obesity). But all these are nothing compared to its natural evolution - if you don't reverse this disease, liver cells start dying. When they die, they are replaced by fibrotic tissue, which does not work, a condition known as cirrhosis.

In both situations, but more in cirrhosis, the liver can't eliminate toxic substances, which get afloat in your body, causing brain and heart damage. Fatty liver has also been linked with an increased rate of liver cancer, which is very lethal.

- *Can I get fatty liver even if I don't drink?*

Yes, you can. It's the most common form of fatty liver disease.

It's been scary over 30 years since non-alcoholic fatty liver disease (NAFLD) was first detected. Yet, the statistics now show that one in four Americans have various stages of this disease. Before NAFLD became known, fatty liver disease was mainly attributed to drinking too much alcohol.

- *Is fatty liver treatable?*

Yes. Almost all stages of liver disease (including steatosis and cirrhosis) are reversible. Your liver has an incredible capacity to regenerate. When you start giving it cues to provide a healthy environment, it can easily burn the fat inside its cells and even replace fibrotic tissue with liver tissue. This will cause weight loss and eliminate toxic substances, reducing or annihilation of diseases such as rashes and certain allergies.

- *How to discover if you have fatty liver disease?*

When a type of fat known as triglyceride accumulates in liver cells, a blockage or backup occurs called steatosis. Generally, there are no obvious symptoms. The most common way for your doctor to detect fatty liver disease is through a blood test. Elevated liver enzymes are the first sign that there may be an issue. Fat retention in the cells is the basic cause of fatty liver disease, but determining what is causing this fat build-up will determine how your doctor treats you.

- *Who is at risk of fatty liver disease?*

Anyone is at risk of developing fatty liver disease. The causes range from malnutrition, exposure to drugs or toxins, and hepatitis C. Those most likely to suffer from this include diabetes, alcoholics, and those suffering from obesity. One of the effects of a more severe case of (FLD) is inflammation of the liver, which can cause a host of other complications in your liver as well as other organs. After determining the presence of elevated enzymes, your doctor may order an ultrasound, and ultimately, an MRI is necessary to have a closer look at the organ. Alcohol consumption may or may not be the cause of this ailment, but a rule of thumb is a measurement of consumption. Less than two drinks per day would indicate a non-alcoholic fatty liver, while two or more alcoholic drinks per day would lead to alcoholic fatty liver disease.

- *What are my chances for recovery treatment?*

If caught early, the chances of recovery are generally positive. This assumption is based on determining what is causing (FLD) to begin with. For example, if alcohol consumption is the cause, simply cutting down considerably or quitting altogether may prevent future complications such as cirrhosis of the liver. On the other hand, if the cause is determined to be metabolic, such as diabetes, then the road to recovery may take a different turn. Diabetes disease causes other complications in the body, such as the fatty liver. This is primarily due to excessively high levels of glucose in the blood. It's impossible to tackle the fatty liver issue until the cause, diabetes, is under control. One of the destructive results of fatty liver is inflammation. One of the most natural ways to fight this is with Omega 3 fish oil. Fish oil is full of fatty acids that work to control and decrease inflammation in the body. Foods with high concentrations of EPA and DHA, fatty acids found in fish oil, have been clinically proven to combat the inflammation that results from fatty liver disease. Omega 3 fish oil has been proven to combat fat build-up in the blood, as evidenced by controlling excessive cholesterol levels. The same fatty acids found in fish oil have proven to fight hepatitis which is inflammation of the liver.

Fatty Liver Complications - Important Facts to Remember

The liver is one of the most vital organs that support almost all other organs in the body. Primarily functioning for metabolism, other significant roles of the liver include detoxification, protein synthesis, and biochemical production that especially aids during digestion through generating bile.

There is no artificial organ or artificial devices that could be used to mimic all liver functions. Thus, a simple malfunction due to disorders or diseases should be given immediate attention. One of these is fatty liver complications.

There are two types of FLD depending **on its cause:**

- AFLD or alcoholic FLD is primarily due to heavy consumption of alcoholic drinks. Alcohol hinders the oxidation of fatty acids in the liver and releases fatty acids from the liver. It slows down the discharge of low-density lipoproteins (LDL) in the bloodstream. Thus, controlling the amount of alcohol intake is the first step to partake.
- NAFLD or non-alcoholic FLD, on the other hand, is caused by several factors. These include a high-fat diet, obesity, diabetes, hyperinsulinemia, and metabolic disorder. Weight and sugar level are the main keywords for such disease. Thus, changing eating habits and getting involved with

daily physical exercises to lose weight are essential to prevent or control it.

These two could lead to complications such as hepatitis and cirrhosis by more than 30 percent possibility.

- Hepatitis is an acute infectious disease that damages the liver caused by the hepatitis A virus (HAV). There is no specific cure for hepatitis; however, it is best advised to have enough rest, refrain from indulging in fatty foods and alcohol, and instead have a well-balanced diet and fluids.
- On the other hand, cirrhosis could kill liver cells and could lead to liver failure. It is characterized by the replacement of liver tissue by fibrosis, scar tissue, and regenerative nodules. Likewise, a healthy lifestyle, especially in diet, should be given importance.
- Other complications include cancer and drug damage. Worst, it could lead to inflammation of the liver called steatohepatitis that. This is a fatal fatty liver complication that could happen to anyone.

Reduction in weight, alcohol consumption and controlled diet for fatty liver coupled with constant exercise are the main fatty liver cures - do these before it is too late!

Fatty Liver Stages

There are many different types of liver disease, but liver damage will progress similarly to any liver disease. It is important to know what happens to your liver at each stage of the progression before complete liver failure. Understanding the progression of liver disease may help you make better health choices.

Your liver is one of the most important organs in your body. It is responsible for detoxifying the blood, aiding food digestion, and storing energy as sugars for later use. But those are only the liver's main functions. There are also about 500 other functions that contribute to your health. When your liver cannot function properly, your whole body will be affected.

Here are the four stages of liver disease.

- *Stage 1: The first sign of liver damage is inflammation*

One of your liver's main functions is to detoxify your blood from toxins found in the food you eat and the products you use. The first sign of liver damage is inflammation. Inflammation in the liver is a sign of your immune system responding to foreign substances, such as too many toxins. This can cause your liver to enlarge.

There are many causes of inflammation. Excess fat in the liver, too many toxins, or viral infection in the liver can make your liver tender and swell up. These conditions might cause inflammation in the liver: non-alcoholic fatty liver; alcoholic fatty liver; and liver hepatitis, including viral hepatitis or autoimmune hepatitis.

You can most of the time feel if your liver is injured when you have stomach pain in the liver area (the upper right area of your abdomen). Sometimes, you will feel the heat in the area. There are some cases where you have no sign of inflammation, such as in the non-alcoholic fatty liver.

Let your doctor know if you have any signs of inflammation. Treating your liver at this stage can help reverse liver damage.

- *Stage 2: Fibrosis is the start of liver scarring*

When you do not treat the inflammation, the inflammation will start to cause the liver to scar. These scar tissues will replace the healthy liver tissue and thus reduce liver function. This entire process is called fibrosis.

When the liver's function drops, toxins and fat will continue their build-up in the liver. Besides preventing the liver from functioning, the scar can block blood flow to the organ.

At this stage, there is still a chance to save your liver through medication and lifestyle management. Your liver has an amazing healing ability; thus, it may still heal from this stage.

- *Stage 3: More severe scarring leads to cirrhosis.*

If you don't treat fibrosis, you are at risk of the next stage called cirrhosis, which is severe scarring of the liver. At this point, the liver can no longer heal itself. It can take a long time to develop cirrhosis, sometimes 20 to 30 years. Unfortunately, this is when people start noticing liver disease because the symptoms are more obvious. Cirrhosis can lead to many complications. Some of the symptoms and complications are: fatigue, or feeling tired; weakness; itching; loss of appetite; weight loss; nausea; bloating of the abdomen from ascites, which is a buildup of fluid in the abdomen; edema—swelling due to a buildup of fluid—in the feet, ankles, or legs; spiderlike blood vessels, called spider angiomas, on the skin; and jaundice, a condition that causes the skin and whites of the eyes to turn yellow.

Cirrhosis can lead to several complications, including liver cancer. The treatment for cirrhosis is to control the progress of the scarring and treat any complications and symptoms caused by cirrhosis.

- *Stage 4: Liver failure*

Your liver has lost all ability to function and unable to heal. Liver failure can be a chronic or acute condition. Acute liver failure strikes fast just in 48 hours as a reaction to poison or a drug overdose. While chronic liver failure developed from cirrhosis may have been going on for years. When you have liver failure, your best option might be a liver transplant.

As liver failure gets worse, it can affect you mentally and physically. You may feel confused and disoriented. You may experience diarrhea, loss of appetite, and lose weight rapidly. Because many other conditions can cause these symptoms, it is hard to diagnose liver failure just from a physical exam.

When you get the diagnosis for liver failure, you will immediately get medical attention to salvage what is left of your liver. If this is not possible, the only option may be a liver transplant.

It is important to have your health checked regularly, as liver disease can be detected during the inflammation stage of fibrosis stages through an ultrasound or X-ray of your stomach. If you are treated successfully at these stages, your liver may have a chance to heal itself and recover.

How To Know What Stage Your Fatty Liver Is

Non-alcoholic fatty liver disease (NAFLD) is the term for a wide range of conditions caused by a fat buildup within the liver cells. It is usually seen in people who are overweight or obese.

A healthy liver should contain little or no fat. Most people with NAFLD only carry small amounts of fat, which doesn't usually cause any symptoms and isn't harmful to the liver. This early form of the disease is known as simple fatty liver or steatosis.

However, just because the simple fatty liver is harmless, **it doesn't mean it is not a serious condition:**

- in some people, if the fat builds up and gets worse, it can eventually lead to scarring of the liver
- as the disease is linked to being overweight or obese, people with any stage of the disease are more at risk of developing a stroke or heart attack

NAFLD is often diagnosed after liver function tests (a type of blood test) produce an abnormal result, and other liver conditions, such as hepatitis, are ruled out.

NAFLD is very similar to alcoholic liver disease, but it is caused by factors other than drinking too much alcohol. The four stages are described below.

- *Stage 1: simple fatty liver (steatosis)*

Hepatic steatosis is stage 1 of the condition. This is where excess fat builds up in the liver cells but is considered harmless. There are usually no symptoms, and you may not even realize you have it until you receive an abnormal blood test result.

- *Stage 2: nonalcoholic steatohepatitis (NASH)*

Only a few people with simple fatty liver develop stage 2 of the condition, called nonalcoholic steatohepatitis (NASH).

NASH is a more aggressive form of the condition, where the liver has become inflamed. Inflammation is the body's healing response to damage or injury and, in this case, is a sign that liver cells have become damaged.

A person with NASH may have a dull or aching pain felt in the top right of their abdomen (over the lower right side of their ribs).

- *Stage 3: fibrosis*

Some people with NASH develop fibrosis, where persistent inflammation in the liver results in fibrous scar tissue around the liver cells and blood vessels. This fibrous tissue replaces some healthy liver tissue, but there is still enough healthy tissue for the liver to function normally.

- *Stage 4: cirrhosis*

At this most severe stage, bands of scar tissue and clumps of liver cells develop. The liver shrinks and becomes lumpy. This is known as cirrhosis.

Cirrhosis tends to occur after the age of 50-60, after many years of liver inflammation associated with the early stages of the disease. People with cirrhosis of the liver caused by NAFLD often also have type 2 diabetes.

The damage caused by cirrhosis is permanent and can't be reversed. Cirrhosis progresses slowly, over many years, gradually causing your liver to stop functioning. This is called liver failure.

FATTY LIVER DIAGNOSIS AND TREATMENT

Are you experiencing a variety of undesirable symptoms that include weight loss and fatigue, as well as overall weakness? Are you feeling tired all of the time? You may have fatty liver disease, an extremely high amount of fat cells growing inside the liver.

Our liver has a significant role in metabolism and other functions such as glycogen storage, decomposition of red blood cells, protein synthesis, hormone production, and detoxification of the body. It is situated over the gallbladder in the right portion of the stomach. Because of these, the liver became high-risked to various diseases.

A five to ten percent accumulation of fats against the liver's total weight could already lead to a certain disease such as the fatty liver. Thus, the diagnosis and treatment at an early stage are crucial since no artificial organ or artificial devices could replace all liver functions.

Diagnosis

Fatty liver disease affects over 50% of the 50 and over-population, with a few of the most common causes being obesity and overly excessive alcohol consumption. This liver disease is very serious but can be reversed with time and the proper diet. Suppose you believe that you have the disease. In that case, you must visit your family doctor to have tests run to determine whether or not you have it and whether or not to make a fatty liver diagnosis.

Once this diagnosis has been made, you can start working on improving your health immediately to reverse the effects of fatty liver disease.

Doctors will test you in a variety of different ways to make a fatty liver diagnosis. First, they will press down gently on your abdomen to see if the area is tender and painful to the touch. Inflammation of the liver is very common and is the number one thing that doctors check to diagnose. Next, they will confirm the results of this 'test' with various blood tests to check the number of fatty cells. Other methods used when making a fatty liver diagnosis are a CT scan, a liver biopsy, or even an ultrasound.

If you are diagnosed with one of the varieties of fatty liver disease, it is essential to know that this disease can be reversed with time. By taking the medications that your doctor provides to you and adhering to a healthy diet, you can begin to reverse the effects of this disease. Being healthy is a number one concern, and it should be treated as such. If diagnosed with this disease, it is up to you to become healthy again!

Without accurate, prompt diagnosis and appropriate care, fatty liver disease can cause liver scarring and permanent, irreversible damage or complete liver failure.

However, because there are often no symptoms, it is not easy to find fatty liver disease. Your gastroenterologist may suspect that you have it if you get abnormal results on liver tests that you had for other reasons.

To make a diagnosis, **your gastroenterologist will use:**

- Your medical history - Questions may be asked regarding alcohol consumption, medication use (both prescription and over-the-counter), and past medical history.
- A physical exam - Physical examination may reveal an enlarged liver palpated or felt in the abdomen below the right rib margin. Otherwise, it may require the development of cirrhosis to elicit abnormalities on physical examination.
- Various tests, including blood and imaging tests, and sometimes a biopsy

Treatment

If the diagnosis is positive, then the treatment of fatty will follow depending on the severity and cause.

- AFLD or alcoholic liver disease is primarily due to heavy consumption of alcoholic beverages because alcohol hinders the oxidation of fatty acids in the liver and the release of fatty acids from the liver as it slows down the discharge of low-density lipoproteins (LDL) in the bloodstream. A person will then be advised to control alcohol level intake and may be advised to refrain drinking alcohol for a faster recovery period.
- On the other hand, NAFLD, or non-alcoholic disease, is caused by several factors such as a high-fat diet, obesity, diabetes, hyperinsulinemia, and metabolic disorder. Weight and sugar level are the main keywords for such disease. Thus, changing eating habits and getting involved with daily physical exercises to lose weight are essential for its treatment. Introducing green-leafy vegetables and fruits

especially rich in vitamin C in your diet will then be advised since these groups aid in digestion and enhance resistance.

Obesity is also one of the main causes of fat accumulation in the liver. Regular exercise such as brisk walking, jogging, swimming, biking, and dancing could stimulate circulation and help flush fats from the liver.

The appropriate treatment for fatty liver disease depends on what is causing it. It is a condition that is reversible if treated at an early stage. People who have this condition have fat in their liver cells. It can be seen in people who ingest a lot of alcohol or people who are obese.

There is not one routine treatment for nonalcoholic fatty liver disease. Doctors work to treat the cause. If the cause is obesity, doctors work with the patient to lose weight through changes in diet, exercise, weight loss surgery, or medications. It is also important to refrain from alcohol.

Alcoholic fatty liver disease is the second type. Symptoms may include weight loss, fatigue, or pain in the upper right stomach. There may be no symptoms at all—the majority of people in the United States who abuse alcohol end up with this condition. The liver ends up enlarged, which causes discomfort. Quitting drinking is the first step of treating the alcoholic version of this disease. Continued alcohol use can lead to advanced diseases. Advanced diseases include alcoholic hepatitis and cirrhosis. Treatments appropriate for this disease caused by obesity are also appropriate for the disease induced by alcohol use.

Eating healthy, losing weight, and exercising are good for both forms of fatty liver disease and overall health. It is important to get routine checkups with a medical doctor because that is the most common way this disease is found. A fatty liver may show up on x-rays or ultrasounds and may be confirmed with a biopsy. After anesthesia, a doctor removes a tiny part of the liver, which is looked at under a microscope. The doctor looks for inflammation, signs of fat, and damage. The diagnosis is fatty liver if inflammation and damage are not present.

Treating fatty liver disease is important because not treating it can cause liver problems to get worse. The liver has many functions that are very important to the body. Here is a list of some of the things the liver does: it produces substances that break down fat, produces cholesterol, filters harmful things from the blood, and makes certain amino acids. That is why it is important to make sure the liver remains healthy.

Fatty liver is a normal condition unless it will reach its extreme condition. Don't wait for it to happen - repair your liver immediately! Diagnose now and treat soon!

Fatty Liver and Diet - Understanding the Relationship to Control FLD

Fatty liver, popularly known as FLD or fatty liver disease, is caused by too much fat accumulation in the liver cells. If such disorder is not given the proper attention and control, it could be fatal in the long run. The good news is that it could be treated and controlled through dietary changes. Thus, having proper knowledge and understanding regarding the link between fatty liver and diet is essential for a person to control such disease.

Our liver has a significant role in metabolism and other functions such as glycogen storage, decomposition of red blood cells, protein synthesis, hormone production, and detoxification of the body. However, due to its location and several functions, the liver is also high-risked to various diseases.

A five to ten percent accumulation of fats against the liver's total weight is already a case of a disease. Before the condition gets severe, fatty liver and diet relationship should be given immediate attention. **A proper diet should be the following:**

- **Low-glycemic diet.** Once the blood sugar rises, the risk of having the disease also increases. Thus, a person should avoid food such as candies, chocolates, concentrated sugars, and other sweets. High-sugar and alcoholic drinks are the main factors for excessive fat accumulation in the liver because they serve as barriers to the oxidation of fatty acids in the liver. Another bad thing is that they slow down the release of low-density lipoproteins (LDL) in the bloodstream, responsible for releasing the fatty acids from the liver.
- **Low-carb diet.** Avoid foods containing simple carbohydrates such as pasta, white bread, and rice. Simple carbohydrates are easily broken down and used by the body quickly. Once the body consumes it, starvation occurs that automatically commands the brain to produce fatty acid in the liver.
- **High-fiber diet.** Green-leafy vegetables and fruits, especially rich in vitamin C, should be included in the diet. These groups do not only aid in digestion but enhance resistance as well. The general rule for fiber intake should be over 20 grams a day and over 30 grams a day for women and men, respectively.

A person suffering from fatty liver disease could then reduce inflammation, decrease liver enzyme levels, reduce insulin resistance and most importantly, decrease fatty acid accumulation in the body only if he or she is determined to understand and apply the relationship between fatty liver and diet.

How to Choose a Healthy Diet Plan for Fatty Liver

If left untreated, the excess buildup of fat can damage your liver. That is why a comprehensive diet plan that consists of healthy liver foods is so important for you. One of the simplest ways to reverse fatty liver disease is eating a balanced liver-friendly diet.

As you probably know, fatty liver is caused by excess fat accumulation in your liver. In its early stages, the fatty liver disease usually has no symptoms. It is often found on a routine blood test.

Although you may not immediately feel the symptoms when too much fat accumulates in your liver, it causes inflammation and swelling. That's when you start noticing the symptoms.

You may feel a dull ache, burning pain, or heaviness in your abdomen as your liver becomes swollen and inflamed. Inflammation and swelling mean your fatty liver is getting worse.

You may also experience other symptoms such as nausea, low-grade fevers, lack of energy, and generally feeling tired and fatigue.

Before Starting Your Liver Diet...

It is important to understand how your liver plays a vital role in your overall health and well-being. The human liver has several functions such as bile production, blood regulation, detoxification, and metabolism.

Your liver helps emulsify fat by breaking down large fat globules into smaller ones, which are then broken down further by enzymes. Your liver helps regulate and maintain your blood sugar levels. It also filters out toxic substances and excretes the toxins in your urine. Lastly, your liver helps metabolize (break down) fats, carbohydrates, and proteins in the foods you eat.

Therefore, it is important to remember that diet is the number one factor in fatty liver disease. It is the key to either healing--or harming--your liver.

Choosing a Healthy Liver Diet Plan

To determine the specific meals to eat each day, **a healthy liver diet plan should give you plenty of choices from each of these food groups:**

- **Eat low-fat or non-fat foods, especially dairy products.** Drink 2% or non-fat milk. Eat low-fat yogurt and cottage cheese. Stay away from high-fat cheeses (for example, use mozzarella instead of cheddar). Instead of high-calorie ice cream, you can enjoy fruit sorbet or frozen yogurt pops.
- **Always include plenty of high-fiber foods such as fruits and vegetables.** Fresh or lightly cooked fruits and vegetables--especially green vegetables and citrus fruits--are the mainstays of a healthy liver diet. Eat plenty of salads and raw or steamed vegetables.
- **Add complex carbohydrates to your diets, such as whole grains and brown rice.** Eating whole wheat bread and crackers is an excellent choice for you. A bowl of bran cereal, hot oatmeal, or shredded wheat with fresh fruit is a great way to start your day right.
- **Although meats are a good source of protein, too much protein in your diet adds more stress to your liver.** Choose seafood, fish, and lean meats, such as chicken or turkey. Avoid red meat and pork (which are high in fat and harder to digest).
- **Your healthy liver diet plan** should also include essential vitamins and minerals.

Take Good Care of Your Liver--Before the Damage Gets Worse

Keep in mind that if you're feeling symptoms, your liver disease may be getting worse instead of better. With the proper treatment, fatty liver disease is completely reversible. That's why there is hope for a complete cure. You can cure fatty liver by choosing--and sticking to--a healthy liver diet plan.

What Foods Should I Eat If I Have A Fatty Liver?

The question, "What foods should I eat if I have a fatty liver?" is one of the first questions people ask when diagnosed with fatty liver disease (FLD). Since the liver is a critical organ that performs over 200 functions, its health is often related to the rest of your body. Everything you consume is processed in the liver before being sent to other areas of your body, so the foods you eat are extremely important for reducing fat in your liver. As they say, "You are what you eat."

Fat consumption should be your primary concern when deciding what foods to eat for fatty liver. Since FLD is caused by too much triglyceride fat building up in your liver tissues, you'll want to stick to a low-fat diet. Fats should make up no more than 30% of your daily caloric intake. Check food labels and be conscious of what you are eating.

High-fat foods to avoid include processed meats such as hot dogs and sausages and meats from high-fat areas such as wings and ribs. Get into the habit of trimming off excess fat before cooking or eating any meats. Whenever possible, opt for lean white meats such as turkey instead of dark meats like beef.

This doesn't mean you can't have a cheeseburger every once in a while, but the more fat you can cut from your diet, the better chance you'll have of reducing fat in your liver and improving your overall health. Cutting down on fatty foods will also help you lose weight, stress the liver, and help add years to your life.

Like any diet, a diet plan for fatty liver is a committed effort that takes willpower and a strong desire to improve your liver health if you want to succeed. FLD patients can struggle with this since the fatty liver is often asymptomatic in its early stages. It's not like a nagging pain that motivates you every day to get rid of it. Get rid of junk foods to remove any temptations that might pull you away from your goal.

Here are some foods you can eat to lower fat in your liver:

- Generous portions of fruits and vegetables, particularly those high in vitamin E, vitamin C, and folate (strawberries, oranges, spinach, broccoli, potatoes, citrus fruits)
- Bran and oatmeal
- Brown rice
- Whole wheat bread
- Lean, white meats (chicken, turkey)
- Whole-grain muffins
- Raw fruit and vegetable juices
- Water (2 liters per day is recommended)
- Salads (use salad dressing sparingly)
- Seafood
- High fiber cereals
- Pasta (avoid egg noodles)

FATTY LIVER DIET FOODS

A LIVER DIET is necessary for anyone who has been diagnosed with fatty liver disease or who may be at risk of developing the disease. Although trying to adopt a new diet can seem overwhelming, the stress can be eased by taking the process step by step. The first thing to take on is learning what foods this diet allows and restricts.

What to Avoid on a Liver Diet

First, several foods should not be consumed while on a fatty liver diet. These are typically foods that are unhealthy for anyone. Here are the major foods to avoid when eating a liver diet to reduce fatty liver disease and symptoms.

Simple carbohydrates are a component of many foods. When these are consumed, the body breaks them down quickly. This makes it possible to store these foods as fat in much greater quantities than other carbohydrates. Foods that are considered simple carbohydrates include milk products, fruit juices, processed grains like white flour and white rice, and any refined sugar or sugar product such as candy and sodas. On a fatty liver diet, these foods should be limited or eliminated from the diet.

Another cause of the disease is eating foods that have a high-fat content. These foods need to be avoided for those who need to reverse or prevent fatty liver when possible. Fatty foods include meats such as beef and pork. Most dairy products, including milk, cheese, and ice cream, also have too much fat to pass a fatty liver diet. Anything fried like French fries or any fast food should not be eaten during a fatty liver diet. Eggs are not a total no-no, but eggs should be consumed infrequently, about once or twice a week, due to the amount of cholesterol they contain.

The Right Foods for a Fatty Liver Diet

With all the foods to avoid, it may seem overwhelming to begin to think about trying a diet. But in reality, there are plenty of delicious and easy to prepare options that will work well within the realms of a healthy diet for the liver.

Low-fat foods loaded with fiber are a top choice for this type of diet since fatty foods are one of the main reasons a person has fatty liver, to begin with. Low fat, high fiber foods include fresh fruits and vegetables, especially broccoli and leafy greens like spinach. These are packed with nutrients and are good for the liver. Other foods that work well for the diet include beans and whole-grain products such as multi-grain bread, brown rice, whole grain pasta, and quinoa.

Although foods that are very low fat and high in fiber should be the main components of a fatty liver diet, other foods can be used. Lean meat such as chicken and turkey is low in fat than beef and pork and can be incorporated into the diet if used in moderation. Skim milk can also be consumed. The key is a balanced diet full of variation so that the diet can be encouraged into a lifestyle and used over a long time.

The Very Best Diet For A Fatty Liver

Fatty liver disease wasn't even known to be an actual illness for some 30 years. Still, currently, almost a third of all Americans are affected by this disease, and it has become the number one liver disease in the country. But this isn't even the bad news; studies and reports show that this disease is still on the rise and will have detrimental effects on transplant programs on a national level. In simple terms, this means that more than 6 million people in America will need liver transplants in the coming years, resulting in a large percentage of these people not receiving the proper treatment.

Experts and doctors have created two categories for causes of fatty livers; one is alcoholic induced, and the other is non-alcoholic. Excessive alcohol consumption leads to damage and cirrhosis of the liver. In contrast, non-alcoholic fatty liver is a result of fat accumulation, better known as triglycerides, in the liver cells. This can lead to inflammation, scarring, cancer, complete liver failure, and eventual death.

Doctors have pinpointed some of the causes of fatty livers, other than alcohol consumption, diabetes, obesity, metabolic syndrome, excessive fat deposits, high levels of fructose, hypertension, a lazy lifestyle, certain medications, and insulin resistance. There is a wide range of factors that can induce fatty liver disease. But the problem is that most people are not well informed about fatty liver, so they do not take this condition seriously.

One of the most important factors is the diet because the diet a person follows can cause and cure a fatty liver. It is important to mention that just because you have a fatty liver doesn't mean that you have the disease. Therefore, following the right diet can drastically reduce the risk of you developing the disease. This simply means that if you do not have the disease, you should look to follow a diet that will help lower the chance of developing it. Either way, the diet is considered the most effective treatment for this condition because doctors cannot find the complete and perfect medication.

There are several food items that you should try to limit in quantity. White bread, white rice, butter, breakfast cereals, fried and fast food, hamburgers, pizzas, and everything of this nature should be immediately removed from your normal diet. Moreover, foods with high cholesterol, glycerin, fat content, and sugar levels should also be ignored because they can increase the damage to the liver.

The important point to remember is that the weight and types of foods you eat both have a major impact on the liver's health, so you need to indulge in physical activities and follow a diet for this. There are certain foods that you should look to consume more of, such as beans, unprocessed grains, whole grain bread, skimmed milk, foods with high protein levels, cinnamon, vegetables, and fruits. Antioxidants are also very important because they improve the health of the liver. Moreover, start having smaller meals with smaller quantities, but a larger number of meals. Follow these simple rules, and you will feel a major difference in the health of your liver.

Fatty Liver Diet - Friend And Foe Foods To Reduce Fat In The Liver

Without a nutrient-rich fatty liver diet in place, it can be complicated to reduce the effects of steatosis and fatty liver disease (FDL). FDL is present in millions of people worldwide, particularly those who suffer from other conditions such as obesity and type 2 diabetes. Although benign and asymptomatic in many patients, if the disease is not regulated and kept under control, it can progress into a life-threatening ailment through cirrhosis, liver cancer, and eventually total liver failure.

The liver is an amazing organ with over 200 functions. It has often been called the body's "chemical factory" and is a built-in, natural filter. It is also a storehouse for fats, vitamins, and minerals and produces up to 24 oz of bile per day.

Bile is important in the emulsification of fat in the intestines. Emulsification refers to the process of breaking down large fat globules into smaller ones. The liver is also the only organ in the human body capable of regeneration. If it shuts down, death can occur within 24 hours.

Is Fat In The Liver Normal?

You may already know excess fat in the body is often stored in adipocytes (fat cells) in areas such as the belly and thighs. So why does fat get into the liver in the first place?

First, it is important to understand fat in the liver accumulates as triglycerides and not as adipocytes. It's perfectly normal for small amounts to show up and be stored in the liver. **Reasons for this include:**

- Fat metabolism occurs mostly in the liver.
- Under some circumstances, such as when a person experiences hypoglycemia, the liver will convert glycogen to fatty acids.
- Fatty acids are converted into energy in the liver when glucose stores (the main energy source for the body) run low.
- Since fat is not water-soluble, lipoproteins carry fatty acids both from and to the liver to be processed.

With all these processes involving fat occurring in the liver, it only makes sense for some fat to be stored there. However, when fat makes up more than 5-10% of the liver by weight, a fatty liver occurs.

Diet plays a key role in reducing a fatty liver. The greatest foe is fat itself. Therefore, high-fat foods should be avoided. Lean cuts of white meat, such as chicken and turkey, should replace fried and/or dark meats such as beef. Alcohol, as well as high sugar fruit juices and energy drinks, should be avoided.

Instead, try to focus a fatty liver diet plan on liver-friendly foods such as fruits and vegetables (greens, leaves, and vitamin C-rich foods) and complex carbohydrates. Complex carbohydrates break down slowly, giving the body a slow, steady source of energy.

Like those found in sweets, simple carbohydrates should be avoided because they break down quickly and are used rapidly by the body. When the body uses these carbohydrates too fast, it then switches to converting protein to energy taxing for the liver. Protein is better used for producing hemoglobin, an important blood component that takes oxygen to cells throughout the body.

Fatty Liver Diet - 7 Tips to Help You Lose the Fat

Fat that collects on the outside of your body can be easily seen. But what about the fat that goes to where you cannot see it or feel it, like your liver?

It can be amazingly simple and easy for you to reduce or even reverse the negative impacts of fatty liver disease (NAFLD) with the right liver diet plan in place.

The best treatment for fatty liver disease is aimed at losing weight. That's because most people with fatty liver are also suffering from being overweight.

Here are 7 Tips to Lose Weight on a Fatty Liver Diet Plan:

- Plan your foods every day.
- Eat a large fresh green salad every day with one of your meals.
- Eat foods high in fiber and complex carbohydrates, such as whole-grain bread, beans, and fiber-rich cereals.
- Detoxify your liver with foods and nutrients such as beans, brown rice, citrus fruits, and green salads.
- Drink water with a squeeze of lemon to cleanse the excess fatty buildup and toxins from your liver.
- Drink a high-quality meal replacement shake to support your diet. It will stabilize your appetite and help you lose excess weight. Make sure it is easy to take with you wherever you go.
- Eat 5 or 6 small meals or snacks a day, rather than 1 or 2 large meals. Smaller meals eaten throughout the day help keep your blood sugar stable and are gentler and easier on your liver.

Above all, make sure you eat foods that you enjoy. Remember to focus on liver-friendly foods: Green leafy vegetables, and food that are rich in vitamin C, and foods that are high in fiber and complex carbohydrates are vital.

Fatty Liver - 3 Ways to Help Treat Fatty Liver Disease

You do not have to stress and panic about solving your fatty liver disease (FLD). If you want to get rid of your liver cells' excess fat and toxins, a healthy diet plan may be all you need to treat the disease.

Many people have been misled into believing there is a magic pill to cure fatty liver; however, truthfully, there is no. When you are suffering from fatty liver, the first thing you need to do is to recognize what is the best treatment.

Although there may be no quick fix to heal this condition, you can lower and even totally remove the built-up fat in your liver. You can use a diet treatment plan designed to stop and even reverse the excess fat building up in your liver and keep enjoying many of the foods you love.

When my daughter was diagnosed with non-alcoholic fatty liver disease (NAFLD), I began searching and learning about possible treatments. I was able to find out much more about how the liver functions. I learned that the liver is a vital organ for metabolizing sugars and fats and cleansing toxins. For example, it produces bile which emulsifies and breaks down larger fat globules into smaller ones which are then reduced by enzymes.

Here are 3 Ways to Help Treat Fatty Liver:

- *Go Easy on Proteins.*

You should avoid eating too much protein because it puts further strain on your liver. Red meat and pork are the worst offenders. Mild proteins like chicken, turkey, and fish are much better for you and gentler on your liver.

- *Take Vitamins and Supplements.*

Supplementing with B-vitamins can reverse mild fatty liver in most common cases. Antioxidants such as vitamins C and E and Magnesium have been shown to protect the liver and help clear the toxic buildup in your liver cells.

- *Get Tested for Insulin Resistance.*

Most patients with FLD also have insulin resistance. Insulin resistance is a pre-diabetic condition. Doctors report that treatment of insulin resistance has improved outcomes in patients who have this disease. You will want to be tested for insulin resistance. Ask your doctor for advice.

Patients with non-alcoholic fatty liver disease are advised to focus on losing weight through dietary changes. Slow and gradual weight loss is the key. A diet plan that helps you lose weight slowly will go a long way in treating your condition.

In order to care for, reverse or even cure fatty liver, you need to recognize that healthy eating habits and daily physical activity will produce the most successful outcome.

THINGS YOU SHOULD KNOW TO REDUCE FAT IN YOUR LIVER

FIRST AND FOREMOST, a fatty liver diet should focus on moderation and balance. A good diet plan for people with fatty liver disease (FLD) isn't much different than a healthy diet for the average person. You want foods with high nutritional value, and you don't want to eat anything in excess.

The overall goal of a fatty liver diet is to reduce fat intake and encourage the body to use up all available calories as energy. In doing so, the excess storage of fats and carbohydrates in the body can be reduced or eliminated.

Many FLD patients are overweight and/or obese, so coupling a good diet with a strong exercise program can help maximize results to reduce fat in the liver. What's good for your liver is almost always good for the rest of your body, so the right diet plan for the fatty liver can improve overall health and not just the health of your liver.

A properly balanced diet for FLD patients will consist of approximately 20-30% protein, 60-70% carbohydrates, and 20-30% fats. Fats should never exceed 30% of the caloric intake.

It's also important to note that carbohydrates should be complex and not simple. Complex carbohydrates include those found in things like whole grains and pasta. Simple carbohydrates are those found in candy and other sweets and should be avoided. These are the carbohydrates that tend to get stored in adipose cells, leading to weight gain.

Vitamins and minerals are also extremely important because they play star roles in things like metabolism, growth, development, hormone creation, and the formation of red blood cells. They can be extremely beneficial, but certain vitamins and minerals can also be extremely harmful if taken in excess.

Things like folate (folic acid), vitamins B1 (thiamine), B2 (riboflavin), B6 (pyridoxine), B12 (cobalamine), manganese, and selenium are all healthy for the liver. The best sources to obtain these vitamins and minerals are fruits and vegetables, particularly greens, leaves, and those rich in vitamin C.

Simple Recipes For Fatty Liver - Excess Liver Fat Doesn't Mean Your Taste Buds Have To Suffer.

Are there simple recipes for fatty liver that are both nutritious and delicious at the same time? If you've been diagnosed with fatty liver disease (FLD), you may think the rest of your life will be resigned to eating foods that taste no better than a mouthful of cardboard. However, that simply isn't the case.

Although specific recipes for reducing fat in your liver can sometimes be hard to find, it's not impossible. And the best news is many are extremely tasty and can help you forget you're eating low-fat foods. After all, foods that are good for you aren't supposed to taste good, right?

Some of the fatty liver diet recipes I've come across include foods like:

- Roast beef mini rolls
- Potato and tuna salads
- Raisin pancakes
- Mexican omelets
- Caribbean shrimp and peas
- Roast chicken and fish with vegetables
- Peach cobbler

Cooking and eating in a way that helps lower fat in the liver doesn't require any unusual or expensive ingredients. You don't have to be a culinary expert. The main goal is to reduce fat consumption to prevent further build-up of triglycerides in the liver.

A good diet plan will also be well balanced to provide your body with ample opportunity to consume all the necessary vitamins and minerals needed to combat liver problems. These include things like folate (folic acid), vitamin B complexes, selenium, vitamin K, sulfur, and manganese, to name a few.

Being diagnosed with FLD doesn't have to be the end of your love of food. You need to be open to eating in a more holistic and health-conscious way. So which recipe will be the first you're going to try?

Fatty Liver Diet Tips

The need for a fatty liver diet is very important when an individual is diagnosed with fatty liver disease. The basic idea behind adopting a specific diet is to reduce the fat in the liver, plain and simple. It offers a better quality of life centered and concentrated on a healthy and fully functioning liver. This disease is a disease that is caused due to the excess of fat in the liver and internal fat that is not visible to you. If a person follows a correct diet for the proper health of the condition, reducing fat is possible but warranted. This diet will slow the progression of and reverse the effects of fatty liver disease. The only point to be kept in mind is to focus on the proper eating habits meant to eliminate the fat in the diet.

A proper fatty liver diet means the reduction of fat in your meals.

Obesity might often be the consequence of this disease; however, this issue can now be handled by incorporating the right eating habits through a strict diet. Moreover, your diet plan must be mapped according to your needs, but fat reduction must be your aim. One of the basic fatty liver diet tips suggests that you read the product's labels before preparing the meal. This is a vital step because after ensuring the low content of fat in a product, you will know what you are eating. On the other hand, if you skip this step, you might probably bring in more fat that will affect your liver. You must keep a close eye on what you eat each day, and adherence to a fatty liver diet plan will do just that.

Fatty liver disease is grouped into stages, starting with the simple fatty liver. After this stage, the formation is observed along with inflammation. If these stages are not treated with proper care and attention focusing on the liver itself, they are likely to develop further complications. This also includes the possibility of the development of liver cancer. A fatty liver is considered asymptomatic; hence, most people do not realize the symptoms and conditions. In order to get a proper diagnosis, it is ideal to rely on the biopsy of the liver. It will give a clear picture of the internal condition of the liver. With the major developments of science, there are quick solutions that can promote healthy living. Implementing a proper and specific proper diet that includes fresh fruits and vegetables can improve the longevity of strong liver and reverse the formation and inflammation of this disease.

A fatty liver diet is extremely important to slow the progression of fatty liver disease.

Due to the internal developments of fat in the liver, the damages are unobserved by patients. When they are admitted for care, they realize that their issue cannot be treated easily to their surprise. This is the very reason that leads to cirrhosis or liver failure. Therefore, in such a critical situation, the sufferer has only one way out. It is the strict adherence to a proper and healthier diet. You are required to avoid all those food items that are not healthy for your liver. If you allow fatty types of food products, then your liver is susceptible to this disease or damaging the liver.

This condition is formed because of various physical conditions ranging from weight constraints, considerable weight gain due to pregnancy, eating improperly, or high alcohol intake. These factors must be treated and dealt with so that the issue does not arise. The fact is that there is no remedy to it; no surgical methods and no medications or prescriptions on the market can reverse or cure the disease. However, this disorder can be reversed by following healthy eating habits through diet and exercise. The food you eat is transmitted through the liver, so if you overlook a healthy food plan, this condition could be imminent. To reverse or prevent the disease, you will need to adopt a proper and specific diet plan.

Leave the planning of a fatty liver diet to the experts for faster recovery.

A proper and specific diet plan is important, but what basic guidelines should you take? Drawing up your diet could end up in failure and prolong your condition. You need a proven fatty liver diet that has been successful for those who have a fatty liver.

Fatty Liver - Top 10 Detox Tips for a Healthy Liver

Fatty liver is a clear sign that your liver is congested and overworked. If your liver is struggling to detoxify your body, these 10 detox tips will help soothe your liver.

A gentle natural detox diet will help take the pressure off this hard-working organ and start optimizing your liver health. A detox diet or program is all about cleansing the body of toxins and other impurities and replacing them with healthy nutrients. Usually, it takes a few days before you notice the positive effects and begin feeling revived.

Start practicing a new way of caring for your liver today. In a week, you may feel like a new person. **You can use these 10 detox diet tips at home:**

- *Start Reversing the Damage.*

A key function of your liver is clearing toxins from your body. When you have fatty liver, that means there is damage to your detoxification system. Sluggish detoxification causes metabolic waste and toxins to build up in your body. To help reverse this, you can add certain nutrients that act at the cellular level to remove the waste and toxins from your body and soothe your liver. You can reverse the damage by restoring natural balance and harmony to your body with an effective fatty liver diet.

- *Limit Harmful Foods.*

Avoid refined carbohydrate foods (especially sugar and white flour), processed and canned foods, high-fat dairy products (especially hard cheese), and junk foods that are full of toxins, low in nutrients, and lack dietary fiber. Limit or stop using artificial sweeteners. Artificial sweeteners can increase the appetite for sweets and carbohydrates.

- *Eat Healthy Foods.*

Start eating more fresh fruits and vegetables, particularly dark leafy greens. Raw and slightly steamed vegetables are best for vitamins and nutrients. Dried beans, brown rice, and whole-grain bread are excellent sources of liver-friendly nutrients and fiber to detoxify your system gently. Try using honey or stevia as a nutritious replacement for sugars. Be careful with fast foods and regularly eat home-cooked meals.

- *Drink Purified Water.*

Use a reputable water filtration system to ensure you have the cleanest possible water. Or you can purchase purified bottled water. Water coming from public water supplies often contains contaminants from old piping and is full of bacteria.

- *Increase Fluid Intake.*

Drink water and freshly squeezed juices to help flush the toxins from your body. If possible, drink only broths, water, juices, and soft-cooked vegetables to treat your body to a liquid diet one day a week. Doing this gives your digestive system a rest, helps cleanse toxins and waste and reduces the burden on your liver.

- *Drink Herbal Teas.*

Teas made from fresh squeezed Lemon, Dandelion root, Ginger, Peppermint, and Spearmint help promote urination and bowel cleansing, which removes trapped viruses bacteria, and toxins from the body. Sweeten with honey or stevia as a replacement for sugar.

- *Treat Constipation.*

Take natural laxatives like bran cereals or psyllium to ensure regular bowel movements and prevent toxins from building up in your digestive tract.

- *Detox Bath.*

A detox bath will help remove toxins from the inside out. Ginger has natural cleansing powers and is a good way to detox your body. Fill the tub with hot water. Add 1/8 cup of either freshly grated ginger root or ground powdered ginger from the spice rack. Soak in the bath for at least 20-30 minutes if you can. The ginger will start to make you sweat, which helps remove the toxins from your body. You may continue to sweat for an hour or so after the bath, which is a good thing because sweating is your body's way of detoxifying from the inside.

- *Reduce Exposure to Toxins.*

Avoid using artificial air fresheners. Start using natural brands of cosmetics, soaps, shampoos, toothpaste, and natural cleaning products.

- *Rest.*

Try to get 6 to 8 hours of sleep every night. Your body heals best when it is at rest. Give yourself at least 10-15 minutes of quiet time, prayer, or meditation daily. Sleep and quiet time allows your body to recuperate and helps keep your mind at ease. Give yourself permission to get the rest you need to heal your liver.

These detox and diet tips will help relieve liver congestion, cleanse toxins, and soothe your liver, especially if it is struggling to detoxify your body. Keep in mind, before embarking on a detox program; you would be wise to check with your doctor. If you have diabetes, kidney disease, or other chronic conditions, you should not try to detox without the supervision of your primary physician.

HOW TO ELIMINATE A FATTY LIVER PROBLEM

A THOROUGH PHYSICAL at your family doctor's office will include an investigation into your liver enzymes. If a report reveals that your liver enzymes are elevated, it could mean a lot of things. One possibility is that you may end up being diagnosed with a Fatty Liver. Physical signs of a fatty liver can also include a distended abdomen, increased fatigue, and difficulty losing weight. A specialist can also palpate a fatty liver and see the liver's fat deposits during a diagnostic ultrasound.

FACTORS THAT COULD HAVE CONTRIBUTED TO YOUR FATTY LIVER CAN include a combination of things. Genetically, you may be predisposed to having a fatty liver, so you can still get this condition no matter how healthy your daily habits are. However, other factors include frequent alcohol intake, a diet full of foods with fat. For example, typical bar foods such as chicken wings, nachos, and french fries can be very bad for a fatty liver. Similarly, any fast food is usually full of fat. Eating a lot of sugar also would not help your condition. Lastly, having no aerobic activity in your life will not help to eliminate any fat in your body.

The ways you can significantly reduce a fatty liver include two significant changes in your daily routine for overweight people. One factor is the introduction of aerobic exercise into your routine, at least 5 days a week. You need to engage in activities between 20 and 45 minutes that will make you sweat and get your heart rate increased. If you have not exercised for a long time, start with a light jog for a minute or two, followed by a fast-paced walk for a minute, then alternating between a jog and a walk. It is helpful to get a heart rate monitor to increase your heart rate to about 60 or 70 percent of your maximum heart rate. Talk to your doctor or another health care professional to figure out your target heart rate.

The other very important factor is changing your diet. Eat five small meals per day rather than three big meals. Eat until you are only 70 percent full rather than being 100 percent or 120 percent full. Eat fruit in between meals, but not more than 4 fruit per day. Stay away from any fried foods or foods with moderate or high fat. Get used to eating more salads if possible.

If you follow the instructions already mentioned, you will notice your weight being reduced considerably over three months. You will also eliminate your fatty liver and become much healthier overall. This is highly recommended as having a fatty liver can lead to diabetes and other complications later on.

. . .

THERE ARE THREE OTHER THINGS THAT CAN GREATLY HELP YOU eliminate your fatty liver. **These include:**

1. **Taking milk thistle daily.** Go to your local health food store and get yourself some milk thistle tablets. Take some daily as directed on the label.
2. **Drinking Chinese Black Tea for a fatty liver.** Go to a Chinese Herbal store and pick yourself up some Black tea with specific ingredients to reduce a fatty liver. Drink two teas per day.
3. **Eat Chia seed daily.** Chia is full of Omega-3's and antioxidants, along with many other nutrients. Chia is amazing for helping to reduce cholesterol, blood sugar, and fat. The most effective proprietary blend of chia on the market today is Mila. Mila has several advantages over other chia brands, **which include the following:**

- It is the only blend of seeds grown in different regions for maximizing a variety of specific nutrients.
- It is the only tested seed.
- It is the only sliced seed. Grinding the seed can lead to a loss of nutrients, and eating the seed whole will not deliver the same amount of nutrients.
- It is the only seed grown within the most nutritious growing region.
- It is the only seed associated with a company whose main goal is to change the health of starving people worldwide. The company helps others who cannot help themselves and is the only company that offers a tested product and ensures its quality is excellent.

If you alter your lifestyle as described above, your chances of eliminating your fatty liver problem are very good. Yes, it may be a challenge the first few weeks to introduce all of these habits, but in only a couple of weeks, you will feel more energetic, and you will be on your way to a new, healthier you.

How to Get Rid of Fatty Liver

If you have fatty liver, you are not alone! It is the most common liver disease in the United States.

Fatty Liver begins as a mild liver condition where fat starts accumulating in your liver cells. This fat buildup usually causes no damage by itself, and there are no symptoms in the early stages.

However, as more fat builds up in your liver cells, it causes inflammation and swelling of your liver. As your liver struggles to get rid of the fatty buildup, you start experiencing symptoms, and it is a sign that a harmful condition is at work in your body. This is when you start noticing the symptoms of fatty liver.

The first signs of liver inflammation and swelling are:

- Nausea
- Stomach pain

- Abdominal burning sensation
- Rashes
- Tiredness and Fatigue
- Headaches

AT FIRST, YOU MIGHT THINK THAT EATING FATTY FOODS CAUSES FATTY liver, but that is not true.

- Your liver plays an important role in the metabolism (break down) of fats. When something goes wrong in this metabolism process, excess fat starts building up in your liver.

- Many health professionals believe that an overgrowth of Candida albicans, a yeast bacteria found in the intestinal tract, may be the root cause of fatty liver disease. Candida is the most common cause of yeast infections in women. If it over-populates your digestive tract, it causes problems with your metabolism.

- Your liver is responsible for storing excess blood glucose (sugar). If your blood sugar is too high, your liver converts the excess sugar into fat and starts accumulating in your liver. It is important to note, Candida thrives on sugar and refined carbohydrates (foods that convert to sugar in your body) and will make you experience intense sugar cravings.

- Your liver is responsible for removing harmful bacteria and toxins from your blood. It also kills germs that enter your body through the intestine. Processing these bacteria, toxins, and germs by your liver produces toxic by-products in your digestive system. When your digestive system is overwhelmed with toxins, your liver is overwhelmed trying to eliminate toxins.

When your liver struggles to get rid of the fatty buildup, you're feeling the overwhelming symptoms of tiredness, fatigue, stomach pain, and low energy. These symptoms of fatty liver are what's keeping you from enjoying your daily life.

- First, if you are overweight, then losing weight is essential. Weight loss is by far the most important treatment. Research shows that people who lose just 9% of their total body weight could reverse fatty liver disease completely.

- Cut down your intake of sugar. Your liver converts excess sugar into fat. Less sugar in your diet means your liver will not have to work as hard converting the sugar into fat.

- Cut down on simple carbohydrates, especially white bread, pasta, and rice. Your liver converts these simple carbohydrates directly into sugar. Then the sugar is converted to fat, which is stored in your liver.

- You can ease the stress on your liver by eating more complex carbohydrates. Eat fiber-rich whole-grain bread, cereals, crackers, and brown rice.

- Eating fresh fruits and vegetables and drinking plenty of water help eliminate the fatty deposits in your liver. This also helps get rid of toxins from your body, and you can start feeling better fast.

- Finally, use natural cleansing foods, herbs, and supplements to detoxify and purify your liver. This helps soothe the inflammation, relieve the swelling, and ease the pain.

SUPPOSE YOU ARE EXPERIENCING INFLAMMATION, SWELLING, AND other symptoms of fatty liver disease. In that case, that means too much fat is accumulating in your liver cells, and your liver is not functioning at full capacity. The good news is, your liver can regenerate new cells and grow healthy new tissue.

. . .

THE SIMPLE TRUTH IS, YOUR LIVER HAS A REMARKABLE POWER TO HEAL. If you are suffering from fatty liver, it is especially important to start caring for your liver now--before the fatty buildup causes more damage to your liver.

Understanding Insulin Resistance

A HORMONE RELEASED BY THE PANCREAS, INSULIN IS DISPERSED INTO the bloodstream in response to elevated blood sugar (glucose) levels. By pushing glucose out of the bloodstream and into the body's cells, insulin keeps blood glucose levels from becoming too elevated. When these cells receive glucose, they convert it to energy. When glucose is not metabolized properly (when the cells are insulin-resistant), energy production is diminished, resulting in fatigue.

INSULIN RESISTANCE PROHIBITS GLUCOSE FROM ENTERING THE CELLS, causing it to accumulate in the blood. To reduce the glucose in the blood, the body signals the pancreas to produce and release more insulin. High blood insulin levels increase triglycerides, which deposit fatty acids in the liver.

BEING OVERWEIGHT, LIVING A SEDENTARY LIFESTYLE, AND EATING A diet rich in sugar and fat all promote insulin resistance. In extreme cases of insulin resistance, diabetes mellitus develops. Approximately 70 percent of people with diabetes have some form of NAFLD, and 5 to 20 percent of people with diabetes have cirrhosis due to NASH. Independent of fatty liver disease, diabetes is believed to be a risk factor for the development of cirrhosis.

Corrective Action

Since some estimates suggest that as many as one in four people with NAFLD may develop the serious liver disease within 10 years, it is important to consider preventative and treatment options. The preferred course of action will depend on each person's fatty liver cause. **Preferred methods include:**

- **Weight loss and exercise** - A diet and exercise program will reduce the amount of accumulated fat in the liver. The most effective diet is high in fiber, vitamins, and minerals while also being low in calories and saturated fat. Safe weight loss must occur slowly, as a loss of more than two pounds a week may accelerate liver disease progression. Regardless of one's current weight, a healthy diet and daily physical activity will reduce inflammation, lower elevated liver enzyme levels and decrease insulin resistance.

- **Diabetes control** - Strict management of diabetes with diet, medications, or insulin lowers blood sugar, which may prevent further liver damage. It may also reduce the amount of accumulated fat in the liver.

- **Cholesterol control** - Controlling elevated levels of

cholesterol and triglycerides with diet, exercise, and cholesterol-lowering medications may help stabilize or reverse nonalcoholic fatty liver disease.

- **Avoid toxic substances** - With NAFLD, especially the more severe NASH version, alcohol elimination is imperative. It is also important to avoid medications and other substances that can cause liver damage. Talk to your doctor about what to avoid.

- **Antioxidants** - Vitamins E and C, alpha-lipoic acid, and N-acetyl cysteine are antioxidants that may reduce liver damage caused by oxidation, a process where unstable oxygen molecules damage cell membranes.

- **Milk Thistle** - Scientific studies suggest that this herb's chief constituent aids in protecting, healing, and repairing the liver. With physician permission, seek a high-quality, highly absorbable milk thistle for best results.

- **Omega-3 fatty acids** - Found primarily in cold-water fish, fish oils, flax and flaxseed oils, and walnuts, omega-3 fatty acids help protect the liver and reduce inflammation.

Due to their close relationship, recovering from a fatty liver is identical to the steps necessary to combat insulin resistance. A commitment to health through instituting lifestyle changes is our nation's best hope for reducing the occurrence of nonalcoholic fatty liver disease.

Reverse Fatty Liver With the Right Diet

Steatosis is the abnormal retention of lipids within a cell. It subsequently leads to a reversible condition called fatty liver disease, which accumulates fat in the liver. Though the disease is not life-threatening, complications may arise if the underlying cause is not resolved. A fatty liver may occur in any age group. However, it frequently involves females more than males.

Fatty liver disease is categorized into two: non-alcoholic and alcoholic fat-so liver. The alcoholic kind is caused by excessive alcohol intake, while the non-alcoholic one may be caused by metabolism disorders or obesity. Metabolic disorders may come in the form of diabetes mellitus and obesity. Other factors include drugs like tamoxifen and methotrexate and nutritional statuses like over nutrition, severe malnutrition, and a starvation diet.

There are different ways to overcome a fat-so liver. The most appropriate would be adhering to a carefully controlled and well-balanced fatty liver disease diet. One good diet for a fatty liver is a diet that promotes weight loss of 1 to 2 pounds per week. For an alcohol-related fatty organ, abstinence from alcohol intake is a must.

. . .

The diet must be continuously taken even after positive results are observed. All the food groups must be included in the diet. However, certain considerations on the amount of saturated fat, carbohydrates, and sugar must be observed. It must be a well-balanced diet and should be taken five to six meals daily.

The best food that a fat liver must-have is low in saturated fats. Sweet foods and those that are rich in carbohydrates must be taken in smaller quantities. Fresh fruits should be eaten instead of sweets, but they too need to be controlled. Early detection may reverse the condition with the proper treatment plan. Correcting the underlying cause must be addressed initially then a well-balanced fatty organ diet must be carefully initiated. The treatment plan must be carefully planned out and should include the most appropriate foods for a fatty organ and the quantities and number of meals per day.

Choosing the Best Diet Plan For Fatty Liver Disease - 3 Things to Consider

Symptoms for Fatty Liver Disease go largely unnoticed. When diagnosed with it, patients become aware that there is no magic cure: no medication or surgery can make it go away. If not treated properly, the liver could progress to cirrhosis or even liver failure. The only known treatment is a specific fatty liver diet plan that fits the requirements to put this disease in remission. Before choosing any of the current diet plans available today, there are a few things to consider before choosing a plan.

HEALTH AND WELLNESS LIFE

. . .

Understand Fatty Liver Diet Plan Requirements

First and foremost, get with your doctor. Doctors will guide you through many different options and educate you with the knowledge to succeed. Fatty Liver Disease happens mostly because of high-glycemic foods in the diet, which raise blood sugar fast. Foods like white bread, white rice, and concentrated sugars contribute to this.

The best foods to switch your diet to involve low-fat diets, diets that are high in fiber, low-calorie, low in saturated fat, with the total fat no more than 30 percent of total calories. Make sure to get a complete understanding of which foods to stay away from and what foods to start implementing into your diet. Most importantly, understand that losing weight too quickly can worsen the disease.

Find Diets that Make Sense

There are thousands of diets on the market today, but few offer customizable plans that match the specifics for FLD. What's more, diets don't have to be boring or lacking taste either. A NAFLD diet doesn't mean you need to become a vegetarian unless you want to do. Some programs give you personal attention, buddy and community systems, will track your progress, and coach you along the way. Popular plans even deliver healthy meals right to your door.

. . .

Take the time to research what the diet plan offers, always ensuring that your plan meets the requirements for treating Fatty Liver Disease.

Make and Keep the Commitment

Not following a specific diet plan for Fatty Liver Disease will worsen and progress the disease, leading to death. Consciously accepting a lifestyle change and owning the commitment is a serious challenge. If you have had trouble dieting in the past, you could get extra help and support with individuals currently fighting the disease. Look online to forums, or your doctor might know some local support groups.

Wellness experts, personal trainers, and life coaches can also be that little extra help and support you need to make the lifestyle change. Remember, these people make a living out of making their clients successful. Dieting is no easy commitment, and you have to be determined and dedicated to your dieting goals.

Ways Everyone (Especially Children) Can Protect Against Fatty Liver

The growing occurrence of non-alcoholic fatty liver disease (NAFLD) has grown increasingly in the last few years. A study estimated that 20% of all Americans had the disease, and now experts think that figure has grown to as high as 33%. The increase in the number of children with the problem indicates that the disease will remain on the increase for many years unless a large-scale change in diet and lifestyle takes place. Obesity is considered the major cause of NAFLD, and obesity in the two to nineteen age group has nearly tripled since 1980.

Since the earliest stages of fatty liver cause few signs or symptoms, why do we consider it such a problem? The condition is broken down into two categories depending on how it was caused: non-alcoholic and alcoholic fatty liver disease. Alcoholic fatty liver is triggered by alcohol abuse, and the problem can often be reversed by giving up alcohol.

Most overweight people, especially in the midsection, begin to form excess fat deposits within the liver. It is seen most often in middle-aged people, more common with women than men and of course with overweight people. It has also been an issue with people who lose weight on a very rapid basis. It is a critical health issue, like a poorly functioning liver can trigger many different health problems, such as additional weight gain, high blood pressure, and type 2 diabetes. About 75% of all those diagnosed with NAFLD have also been found to have type 2 diabetes.

If you or your child is fighting obesity problems, **there are five lifestyle changes you can make to reverse the problem:**

- **Exercise.** Studies show that you don't have to train like an athlete to boost your liver health. Certainly, the more exercise you can do them better, but anything you do to break up the sedentary time will be beneficial. So, between television shows, go out, take a brisk, ten-minute walk, or if the weather is bad, do some jumping jacks or a short yoga session.

- **Snack on loads of produce.** Too much fructose, even in the form of fruit, is not completely healthy. But the fiber, antioxidants, and enzymes in fruit will always make it a better snack alternative than candy or chips. Vegetables usually aren't as sweet on the palate, but a low-fat veggie dip is really good and perhaps the healthiest option of all.

- **Portion sizes.** Even when you eat the right foods, you will battle weight if your portion sizes are too large. For the most part, restaurants look as they're providing value super-size everything, but they do us no favors. Develop a clock in your brain that tells you when to stop eating, and take the rest home for another meal.

- **Liver-friendly foods.** Certain foods, often in the spice and herb category, are especially good for the liver. Milk thistle and curcumin (found in turmeric) are two, but many others explore.

- **Carbonated beverages.** These have been a staple in the western diet, but the high levels of fructose and chemical sweeteners make them poison to the system.

Fatty Liver Disease Treatment - Three Supplements to Cure Your Liver

You have followed the advice about diet and exercise and how it applies to curing liver disease, and you started to see results. You now understand how getting rid of fatty liver can change your life, but you want to get there faster.

What do you do?

Here are the three supplements all studies agree will regenerate your liver. And you don't need to be skeptical about them - they were tested in scientific studies and reversed not only mild cases of liver disease but even liver cancer and failure. So much so that the pharmaceutical industry is already performing various studies to extract the active substance from them and create a new liver pill.

- *Ginger*

Ginger is an excellent addition to your kitchen. It has a spicy flavor (be careful not to add too much), and you can find it dried, fresh, and pickled. You can use it as a condiment or make tea with it (try ginger and lemon tea). Pickled ginger is used to reset your tongue between two different flavored dishes, so the flavor from the first doesn't taint the second flavor.

GINGER IS ALSO USED IN GINGERBREAD, COOKIES, CAKES, GINGER ALE, ginger beer... However, the other substances in these recipes are not very good for your liver, and you should avoid them.

- *Turmeric*

YET ANOTHER POWERFUL CONDIMENT. TURMERIC BELONGS TO THE ginger family, and its main use is in curries to impart rich yellow color. It is also used for this purpose in several dairy and baked products.

FRESH TURMERIC IS HARD TO COME BY. IT CAN BE USED TO MAKE pickles or added to salads. Its leaves are traditionally used in Ayurvedic practices.

- *Milk Thistle*

THIS IS THE HOLY GRAIL OF LIVER-PROTECTING SUPPLEMENTS - IT CAN even cure acute cases of mushroom poisoning that would otherwise kill a person. It is already used for this purpose by Western medicine at hospitals.

. . .

IT CAN EASILY BE FOUND IN CAPSULES, BUT IT CAN ALSO BE USED IN salads and even roasted if you can find it fresh. It is closely related to the artichoke, and a few studies have shown that the artichoke has liver healing properties, so you may want to add it to your diet.

WEIGHT LOSS FOR FATTY LIVER DISEASE

LOSING weight is a slow and difficult process for most people. However, for individuals with a fatty liver, it is even more challenging. Fatty liver is an extremely common problem that affects approximately one in five people. If you carry excess abdominal weight, you probably have a fatty liver yourself; your doctor just hasn't diagnosed it yet.

One of the liver's main jobs is to burn off excess body fat and get rid of it through the gallbladder and out in bowel motions. Unfortunately, a fatty liver cannot achieve this task very well. A fatty liver is doing the opposite of what it should be – it is accumulating fat. Luckily there are several ways to overcome this obstacle and achieve weight loss.

People with a fatty liver have a slow metabolic rate. They usually also suffer from syndrome X (metabolic syndrome/insulin resistance), and they often have a sluggish thyroid gland. Combine that with fatigue and poor sleep, and you can see how it becomes almost impossible to stick to a healthy diet and exercise plan.

Here are some of the tips for getting your liver to burn fat again:

- **Reduce the sugar, carbohydrate, and bad fats in your diet.** These foods are what creates a fatty liver in the first place. Most people with a fatty liver got one because they ate more carbohydrates than their liver could process. Carbohydrate-rich foods include sugar, flour, bread, pasta, rice, potatoes, breakfast cereals, and grains. The liver is very proficient at converting these foods into fat. The other food that promotes the formation of a fatty liver is omega 6 rich vegetable oil. Fried foods and packaged foods like crisps, chips, crackers, and cookies are usually full of the wrong fats.
- **Base your diet on vegetables, protein, and good fats.** These foods will keep you feeling full and will keep your blood sugar level stable throughout the day. This is very important to prevent hypoglycemia, sugar cravings, foggy head, and fatigue. Many people trying to lose weight don't eat enough protein and fat. They are in such a rush to lose weight and want to reach their goal tomorrow to eat too little food. This is dangerous territory because you will be at far greater risk of binging on all the wrong foods once you get tired and hungry enough. When eating protein-rich foods like fish, poultry, or red meat, please eat a palm and a half-sized portion. Whey protein powder is an excellent source of protein that's highly satiating. It will help to keep you feeling full for many hours and reduces the risk of sugar cravings. Please include good fats in your diets like olive oil, avocados, nuts, seeds, and oily fish such as salmon. People who don't eat enough protein and fat usually crave sugar and carbohydrate.
- **Take a good quality liver tonic.** Diet changes will work

on their own eventually, but you should reach your goal weight sooner and feel more energetic sooner if you take a good quality liver tonic. Livatone Plus contains the nutrients your liver needs to burn fat efficiently and detoxify your bloodstream.

- **Check if you have diabetes or syndrome X.** Type 2 diabetes is a rapidly growing disease, and approximately half of the people who have it don't realize it because they haven't been diagnosed yet. See your doctor and ask for a fasting blood glucose test to check if you have diabetes. Syndrome X is even more common. If you have a large waist, then you have syndrome X. If you have a more advanced case of syndrome X, you have high blood pressure, high blood triglycerides, good low cholesterol (HDL), and bad high cholesterol (LDL). Diabetes and syndrome X make weight loss extremely difficult because of the elevated blood insulin, which is a feature of these conditions. The herbs and nutrients in Glycemic Balance capsules help to lower insulin, thereby making weight loss easier.
- **Eat more raw vegetables.** No matter where you live, it is important to eat raw food such as salad every day. Try to eat as many different colored vegetables as possible because the pigments in vegetables are antioxidants, and they each have unique benefits. Your liver and bowels need the nutrients in raw vegetables to function at their optimum. It is well worth adding raw juices to your diet.

Weight loss takes more time and commitment for those with a fatty liver, but with the right technique, it is achievable.

Fatty Liver Diet - A 1200 Calorie Diet Plan That Works To Shed Weight And Reduce Fat In The Liver

A fatty liver diet should focus on shedding pounds and reducing excess fat in the body. By reducing excess fat consumption, the opportunity for fat congestion in the liver is greatly reduced. It is generally recommended that people with fatty liver disease (FLD) follow a 1200 to 1500 calorie diet. No more than 30% of the calories should be composed of fat.

To explain this more tangibly, we can do a little bit of math to figure out how many grams of fat you should be consuming each day. If no more than 30% of a 1200 calorie diet is to be made up of fat, that means no more than 360 calories should be fat (1200 calories x 0.30 = 360).

One gram of fat is equivalent to 9 calories. Therefore, no more than 40 grams of fat should be consumed each day (360 calories/9 calories per gram = 40 grams).

A 1200 to 1500 calorie diet should target high amounts of complex carbohydrates with little protein and fat. A diet such as this can help FLD patients lose as much as 2lbs per week. **Here is how this diet should be broken down:**

- 6 ounces of protein (stick to lean white meats such as fish, turkey, and chicken or get protein from vegetable sources such as beans)
- 4 or more servings of vegetables (greens, leaves, legumes, or others high in folate)
- 3 servings of fruits (citrus fruits high in vitamin E and vitamin C are recommended)
- 5 servings from foods high in starch such as potatoes or whole-grain bread
- 3 servings of fat (try to stay away from saturated fats and instead opt for unsaturated fats in limited quantities)

- 2 servings of dairy (focus on low-fat and non-fat alternatives)

It's important not to miss any meals. Calories should be broken down and consumed throughout the day. For example, 300 calories for breakfast, 100 calories for a morning snack, 300 calories for lunch, 50 calories for an afternoon snack, and 450 calories for dinner.

These numbers serve only as a guideline and are not set in stone. You may find it easier to eat less for breakfast, lunch, and dinner and have a few more little snack times throughout the day.

The important part of this diet plan for fatty liver is not exceeding the 1200 to 1500 calories per day limit. Eat small meals regularly rather than one huge meal all at once to keep your body from going into starvation mode and producing fatty acids that can lead to further fat congestion in the liver. For the same reason, strive for gradual weight loss of a pound or 2 per week rather than trying to shed dozens of pounds at once.

Many diet recipes for fatty liver exist that will keep your taste buds from getting bored.

Exercise for Fatty Liver Disease

Fatty liver is the build-up of fat in liver cells. It usually is caused by obesity but may also result from diabetes, high triglycerides, and, in some cases, alcohol abuse, rapid weight loss, malnutrition, and long-term use of certain medications.

The danger of fatty liver is that it can lead to localized inflammation, which can progress to a condition called NASH (Non-Alcoholic Steatohepatitis). (If alcohol abuse is involved, the condition is termed "alcoholic steatohepatitis"). NASH can cause scarring and hardening of the liver, leading to cirrhosis, a very serious disease, and liver cancer.

The only ways to deal with fatty liver are losing weight and lowering your triglycerides if they're elevated. If you have diabetes, the focus should be to make sure that your diabetes and weight are well controlled. Regular exercise is important since it can help you lose weight. Still, new research suggests that resistance training may be an effective way to reduce fatty liver just as aerobic activity is, even if you don't lose much weight.

Here are some of the exercises you can go with:

- Aerobic
- Interval (Anaerobic) Training
- Strength Training
- Core Exercises

Fatty Liver - The Truth About Olive Leaf Extract to Reduce Fatty Liver

How can a little glossy green olive leaf reduce fatty liver? Because a natural substance in olive leaf extract can lower your blood sugar. And lowering your blood sugar may be the most important way to reduce fatty liver naturally. At least, that's what some researchers say.

Let me explain. Specifically, olive leaf extract has been tested and shown to contain a powerful natural ingredient that can reduce blood sugar and reduce fatty liver.

Olive Leaf Extract

Olive leaf extract is a natural compound extracted from olive tree leaves. Olive leaves are widely used as remedies in Europe and

Mediterranean countries, where herbal extracts, powders, and teas, are traditionally prescribed as effective forms of treatment.

You can find natural supplements that contain olive leaf extract in most drug stores or pharmacies.

Control Blood Sugar

Results of a clinical study reported suggest olive leaf extract can control the level of sugar in your blood:

The clinical study tested 79 adults with Type 2 Diabetes. The U.S. National Library of Medicine defines type 2 diabetes as "a lifelong (chronic) disease in which there are high levels of sugar (glucose) in the blood." Type 2 diabetes is commonly found in people who have fatty liver disease.

In the study, some participants took a supplement that contained olive leaf extract while others in the group took a placebo. Researchers gave the participants olive leaf extract in 500 mg oral tablet form daily for 14 weeks.

At the end of the study, the test results showed marked improvements in people who took the supplement. They had a remarkable drop in their blood sugar levels (compared to participants in the placebo group) and maintained more stable glucose levels.

The researchers concluded that olive leaf extract may be an effective adjunct therapy that normalizes glucose homeostasis in individuals with diabetes. In short, "homeostasis" is the ability of a body to maintain internal stability and metabolic equilibrium.

In other words, this powerful supplement looks promising to keep your blood sugar under control--which is the most important factor to reduce your fatty liver naturally.

Reduce Fatty Liver

A researcher in nutrition and metabolism confirmed that:

Non-alcoholic fatty liver disease is a metabolic syndrome that is strongly associated with poor blood sugar control.

- Common sugar-related problems linked to the fatty liver are: High blood sugar
- Type 2 Diabetes
- Weight gain
- Insulin resistance
- Slow metabolism

Researchers say olive leaves contain "several bioactive compounds" with the potential to reduce and regulate blood sugar levels.

These medical reports show incredible potential for people who want to take care of their liver. Now you know more about what you can do to take care of your liver, too. Imagine the relief when that dull, heavy ache in your swollen liver is gone.

It's clear; evidence shows the little green olive leaf may be powerful enough to lower your blood sugar and reduce fatty liver naturally.

Fatty Liver Diet Meal Plan

You must begin changing your eating habits if you want to avoid fibrosis and cirrhosis (end-stage, advanced scarring of the liver). Do not be afraid if you have fatty liver - it's not the end of your life!

By simply changing how you cook and eat, you will be able to reverse the effects of a lifetime of bad eating habits. Liver health begins with what we eat. **Below are some recipes to start changing your life:**

Day 1: Monday

Breakfast: Banana Yogurt Pots

Macros:

- Calories – 236
- Protein – 14g
- Carbs – 32g
- Fat – 7g

Prep time: 5 minutes

Ingredients (for 2 people)

- 225g / ⅞ cup Greek yogurt
- 2 bananas, sliced into chunks
- 15g / 2 tbsp walnuts, toasted and chopped
- Instructions
- Place some of the yogurts into the bottom of a glass. Add a layer of banana, then yogurt, and repeat. Once the glass is full, scatter with the nuts.

Lunch: Cannellini Bean Salad

Macros:

- Calories – 302
- Protein – 20g
- Carbs – 54g
- Fat – 0g

Prep time: 5 minutes

Ingredients (for 2 people)

- 600g / 3 cups cannellini beans
- 70g / ⅜ cup cherry tomatoes, halved

- ½ red onion, thinly sliced
- ½ tbsp red wine vinegar
- small bunch basil, torn

Instructions

- Rinse and drain the beans and mix with the tomatoes, onion, and vinegar. Season, then add basil just before serving.

Dinner: Moussaka

Macros:

- Calories – 577
- Protein – 27g
- Carbs – 46g
- Fat – 27g

Prep time: 30 minutes

Ingredients (for 2 people)

- 1 tbsp extra virgin olive oil
- ½ onion, finely chopped
- 1 garlic clove, finely chopped
- 250g / 9 oz lean beef mince
- 200g can / 1 cup chopped tomatoes
- 1 tbsp tomato purée
- 1 tsp ground cinnamon
- 200g can / 1 cup chickpeas
- 100g pack / ⅔ cup feta cheese, crumbled
- Mint (fresh preferable)
- Brown bread, to serve

Instructions

- Heat the oil in a pan. Add the onion and garlic and fry until soft. Add the mince and fry for 3-4 minutes until browned.
- Tip the tomatoes into the pan and stir in the tomato purée and cinnamon, then season. Leave the mince to simmer for 20 minutes. Add the chickpeas halfway through.
- Sprinkle the feta and mint over the mince. Serve with toasted bread.

Day 2: Tuesday

Breakfast: Tomato and Watermelon Salad

Macros:

- Calories – 177
- Protein – 5g
- Carbs – 13g
- Fat – 13g

Prep time: 5 minutes

Ingredients (for 2 people)

- 1 tbsp olive oil
- 1 tbsp red wine vinegar
- ¼ tsp chilli flakes
- 1 tbsp chopped mint
- 120g / ⅝ cup tomatoes, chopped
- ½ watermelon, cut into chunks
- 50g / ⅔ cup feta cheese, crumbled

Instructions

- For the dressing, Mix the oil, vinegar, chilli flakes, and mint, and then season.
- Put the tomatoes and watermelon into a bowl. Pour over the dressing, add the feta, then serve.

Lunch: Edgy Veggie Wraps

Macros:

- Calories – 310
- Protein – 11g
- Carbs – 39g
- Fat – 11g

Prep time: 10 minutes

Ingredients (for 2 people)

- 100g / ½ cup cherry tomatoes
- 1 cucumber
- 6 Kalamata olives
- 2 large wholemeal tortilla wraps
- 50g / ¼ cup feta cheese
- 2 tbsp hummus

Instructions

- Chop the tomatoes, cut the cucumber into sticks, split the olives, and remove the stones.
- Heat the tortillas.
- Spread the houmous over the wrap. Put the vegetable mix in the middle and roll-up.

Dinner: Spicy Tomato Baked Eggs

Macros:

- Calories – 417
- Protein – 19g
- Carbs – 45g
- Fat – 17g

Prep time: 25 minutes

Ingredients (for 2 people)

- 1 tbsp olive oil
- 2 red onions, chopped
- 1 red chili, deseeded & chopped
- 1 garlic clove, sliced
- small bunch coriander stalks and leaves chopped separately
- 800g can / 4 cups cherry tomatoes
- 4 eggs
- brown bread, to serve

Instructions

- Heat the oil in a frying pan with a lid, then cook the onions, chili, garlic, and coriander stalks for 5 minutes until soft. Stir in the tomatoes, then simmer for 8-10 minutes.
- Using the back of a large spoon, make 4 dips in the sauce, then crack an egg into each one. Put a lid on the pan, then cook over low heat for 6-8 mins, until the eggs are done to your liking. Scatter with the coriander leaves and serve with bread.

Day 3: Wednesday

Breakfast: Blueberry Oats Bowl

Macros:

- Calories – 235
- Protein – 13g
- Carbs – 38g
- Fat – 4g

Prep time: 10 minutes

Ingredients (for 2 people)

- 60g / ⅔ cup porridge oats
- 160g / ⅗ cup Greek yogurt
- 175g / ¾ blueberries
- 1 tsp honey

Instructions

- Put the oats in a pan with 400ml of water—heat and stir for about 2 minutes. Remove from the heat and add a third of the yogurt.
- Tip the blueberries into a pan with honey and 1 tbsp of water. Gently poach until the blueberries are tender.
- Spoon the porridge into bowls and add the remaining yogurt and blueberries.

Lunch: Carrot, Orange, and Avocado Salad

Macros:

- Calories – 177
- Protein – 5g

- Carbs – 13g
- Fat – 13g

Prep time: 5 minutes

Ingredients (for 2 people)

- 1 orange, plus zest and juice of 1
- 2 carrots, halved lengthways, and sliced with a peeler
- 35g / 1 ½ cups rocket / arugula
- 1 avocado, stoned, peeled, and sliced
- 1 tbsp olive oil

Instructions

- Cut the segments from 1 of the oranges and put them in a bowl with the carrots, rocket/arugula, and avocado. Whisk together the orange juice, zest, and oil. Toss through the salad and season.

Dinner: Salmon with Potatoes and Corn Salad

Macros:

- Calories – 479
- Protein – 43g
- Carbs – 27g
- Fat – 21g

Prep time: 30 minutes

Ingredients (for 2 people)

- 200g / 1 ⅓ cups baby new potatoes

- 1 sweetcorn cob
- 2 skinless salmon fillets
- 60g / ⅓ cup tomatoes
- 1 tbsp red wine vinegar
- 1 tbsp extra-virgin olive oil
- Bunch of spring onions/scallions, finely chopped
- 1 tbsp capers, finely chopped
- handful basil leaves

Instructions

- Cook potatoes in boiling water until tender, adding corn for the final 5 minutes. Drain & cool.
- For the dressing, mix the vinegar, oil, shallot, capers, basil & seasoning.
- Heat grill to high. Rub some dressing on salmon & cook, skinned side down, for 7-8 minutes. Slice tomatoes & place them on a plate. Slice the potatoes, cut the corn from the cob & add to the plate. Add the salmon & drizzle over the remaining dressing.

Day 4: Thursday

Breakfast: Banana Yogurt Pots

Lunch: Mixed Bean Salad

Macros:

- Calories – 240
- Protein – 11g
- Carbs – 22g
- Fat – 12g

Prep time: 10 minutes

Ingredients (for 2 people)

- 145g / ⅘ cup jar artichoke heart in oil
- ½ tbsp sundried tomato paste
- ½ tsp red wine vinegar
- 200g can / 1 cup cannellini beans, drained and rinsed
- 150g / ¾ cup tomatoes, quartered
- handful Kalamata black olives
- 2 spring onions, thinly sliced on the diagonal
- 100g / ⅔ cup feta cheese, crumbled

Instructions

- Drain the jar of artichokes, reserving 1-2 tbsp of oil. Add the oil, sun-dried tomato paste, and vinegar and stir until the smooth—season to taste.
- Chop the artichokes and tip into a bowl. Add the cannellini beans, tomatoes, olives, spring onions, and half of the feta cheese. Stir in the artichoke oil mixture and tip into a serving bowl. Crumble over the remaining feta cheese, then serve.

Dinner: Spiced Carrot and Lentil Soup

Macros:

- Calories – 238
- Protein – 11g
- Carbs – 34g
- Fat – 7g

Prep time: 25 minutes

Ingredients (for 2 people)

- 1 tsp cumin seeds
- pinch chilli flakes
- 1 tbsp olive oil
- 300g /2 cups carrots, washed and coarsely grated
- 70g / ⅓ cup split red lentils
- 500ml / 2 ¼ cups hot vegetable stock
- 60ml / ¼ cup milk
- Greek yogurt, to serve

Instructions

- Heat a large saucepan and dry fry the cumin seeds and chilli flakes for 1 minute. Scoop out about half of the seeds with a spoon and set them aside. Add the oil, carrot, lentils, stock, and milk to the pan and bring to the boil. Simmer for 15 minutes until the lentils have swollen and softened.
- Whizz the soup with a stick blender or in a food processor until smooth—season to taste and finish with a Greek yogurt doll and a sprinkling of the reserved toasted spices.

Day 5: Friday

Breakfast: Tomato and Watermelon Salad

Lunch: Panzanella Salad

Macros:

- Calories – 452
- Protein – 6g
- Carbs – 37g

- Fat – 25g

Prep time: 10 minutes

Ingredients (for 2 people)

- 400g / 2 cups tomatoes
- 1 garlic clove, crushed
- 1 tbsp capers, drained and rinsed
- 1 ripe avocado, stoned, peeled, and chopped
- 1 small red onion, very thinly sliced
- 2 slices of brown bread
- 2 tbsp olive oil
- 1 tbsp red wine vinegar
- small handful basil leaves

Instructions

- Chop the tomatoes and put them in a bowl. Season well and add garlic, capers, avocado, and onion. Mix well and set aside for 10 minutes.
- Meanwhile, tear the bread into chunks and place it in a bowl. Drizzle over half of the olive oil and half of the vinegar. When ready to serve, scatter tomatoes and basil leaves and drizzle with remaining oil and vinegar. Stir before serving.

Dinner: Med Chicken, Quinoa, and Greek Salad

Macros:

- Calories – 473
- Protein – 36g
- Carbs – 57g

- Fat – 25g

Prep time: 20 minutes

Ingredients (for 2 people)

- 100g / ⅗ cup quinoa
- ½ red chili, deseeded and finely chopped
- 1 garlic clove, crushed
- 2 chicken breasts
- 1 tbsp extra-virgin olive oil
- 150g / ¾ cup tomatoes, roughly chopped
- handful pitted black kalamata olives
- ½ red onion, finely sliced
- 50g / ½ cup feta cheese, crumbled
- small bunch mint leaves, chopped
- juice and zest ½ lemon

Instructions

- Cook the quinoa following the pack instructions, then rinse in cold water and drain thoroughly.
- Meanwhile, toss the chicken fillets in olive oil with some seasoning, chili, and garlic. Lay in a hot pan and cook for 3-4 minutes on each side or until cooked through. Transfer to a plate and set aside
- Next, tip the tomatoes, olives, onion, feta, and mint into a bowl. Toss in the cooked quinoa. Stir through the remaining olive oil, lemon juice, and zest, and season well. Serve with the chicken on top.

Day 6: Saturday

Breakfast: Blueberry Oats Bowl

Lunch: Quinoa and Stir-Fried Veg

Macros:

- Calories – 473
- Protein – 11g
- Carbs – 56g
- Fat – 25g

Prep time: 30 minutes

Ingredients (for 2 people)

- 100g / ⅗ cup quinoa
- 3 tbsp olive oil
- 1 garlic clove, finely chopped
- 2 carrots, cut into thin sticks
- 150g / 1 ⅔ leek, sliced
- 1 broccoli head, cut into small florets
- 50g / ¼ cup tomatoes
- 100ml / ¼ cup vegetable stock
- 1 tsp tomato purée
- juice ½ lemon

Instructions

- Cook the quinoa according to pack instructions. Meanwhile, heat 3 tbsp of the oil in a pan, then add the garlic and quickly fry for 1 minute. Throw in the carrots, leeks, and broccoli, then stir-fry for 2 minutes until everything is glistening.
- Add the tomatoes, mix the stock and tomato purée, then add to the pan—cover and cook for 3 minutes. Drain the quinoa and toss in the remaining oil and lemon juice.

Divide between warm plates and spoon the vegetables on top.

Dinner: Grilled Vegetables with Bean Mash

Macros:

- Calories – 314
- Protein – 19g
- Carbs – 33g
- Fat – 16g

Prep time: 40 minutes

Ingredients (for 2 people)

- 1 pepper, deseeded & quartered
- 1 aubergine, sliced lengthways
- 2 courgettes, sliced lengthways
- 2 tbsp olive oil
- For the mash
- 400g / 2 cups haricot beans, rinsed
- 1 garlic clove, crushed
- 100ml / ½ cup vegetable stock
- 1 tbsp chopped coriander

Instructions

- Heat the grill. Arrange the vegetables over a grill pan &brush lightly with oil. Grill until lightly browned, turn them over, brush again with oil, then grill until tender.
- Meanwhile, put the beans in a pan with garlic and stock. Bring to the boil, then simmer, uncovered, for 10 minutes. Mash roughly with a potato masher.

Divide the vegetables and mash between 2 plates, drizzle over the oil and sprinkle with black pepper and coriander.

Day 7: Sunday

Breakfast: Banana Yogurt Pots

Lunch: Moroccan Chickpea Soup

Macros:

- Calories – 408
- Protein – 15g
- Carbs – 63g
- Fat – 11g

Prep time: 25 minutes

Ingredients (for 2 people)

- 1 tbsp olive oil
- ½ medium onion, chopped
- 1 celery sticks, chopped
- 1 tsp ground cumin
- 300ml / 1 ¼ cups hot vegetable stock
- 200g can / 1 cup chopped tomatoes
- 200g can / 1 cup chickpeas, rinsed and drained
- 50g / ¼ cup frozen broad beans
- zest and juice ½ lemon
- coriander & bread to serve

Instructions

- Heat the oil in a saucepan, then fry the onion and celery for

10 minutes until softened. Add the cumin and fry for another minute.
- Turn up the heat, then add the stock, tomatoes, chickpeas, and black pepper. Simmer for 8 minutes. Add broad beans and lemon juice and cook for a further 2 minutes. Top with lemon zest and coriander.

Dinner: Spicy Mediterranean Beet Salad

Macros:

- Calories – 548
- Protein – 23g
- Carbs – 58g
- Fat – 20g

Prep time: 40 minutes

Ingredients (for 2 people)

- 8 raw baby beetroots, or 4 medium, scrubbed
- ½ tbsp sumac
- ½ tbsp ground cumin
- 400g can / 2 cups chickpeas, drained and rinsed
- 2 tbsp olive oil
- ½ tsp lemon zest
- ½ tsp lemon juice
- 200g / ½ cup Greek yogurt
- 1 tbsp harissa paste
- 1 tsp crushed red chilli flakes
- mint leaves, chopped, to serve

Instructions

- Heat oven to 220C/200C fan/ gas 7. Halve or quarter beetroots, depending on size. Mix spices together. On a large baking tray, mix chickpeas and beetroot with the oil. Season with salt & sprinkle over the spices. Mix again. Roast for 30 minutes.
- While the vegetables are cooking, mix the lemon zest and juice with the yogurt. Swirl the harissa through and spread into a bowl. Top with the beetroot & chickpeas, and sprinkle with the chilli flakes & mint.

How to Incorporate Fatty Liver Disease Recipes Into Your Treatment

The fatty liver disease presents itself in two ways: alcoholic fatty liver disease and nonalcoholic fatty liver disease or NAFLD. The former occurs in those who abuse alcohol and the latter in those who rarely, if ever, drink alcohol. The disease itself is more than the normal amount of fat within the liver--some fat is normal and normally does not cause a problem.

However, when NAFLD is present, it can lead to serious complications if inflammation and/or scarring occur in the liver. Although there is no specific treatment for this liver disease, the potential contributing factors are treated, such as obesity. Losing weight is recommended, and there are specific fatty liver disease recipes for this purpose.

When diagnosed with this disease and overweight, the doctor will recommend a change in eating habits and suggest incorporating an exercise program into your daily routine. The best exercise to lose weight is cardiovascular exercise (i.e., walking, swimming, or bike riding). The recipes themselves will need to consist of foods of healthy food choices such as fruits and vegetables. These diet recipes should also be low in saturated fats and high in whole grains.

Typical items within these recipes are brown rice, whole wheat bread, certain fish, and nuts. When cooking or choosing a dressing for your salad, you should substitute oils high in saturated fat for olive oil. A fatty liver diet plan should also include lean meats like poultry and avoid red meat whenever possible, as it tends to contain too much unhealthy fat. Carbohydrate and sugar intake should be monitored and kept to a minimum. Not to say to exclude any particular types of carbohydrate but rather your meals should be well-balanced and include all the food groups.

By eating fatty liver disease recipes, doing 30 minutes or more of exercise at least 5 times a week, taking any prescribed medications, and following other doctor orders, you will lose weight and possibly reverse the fatty liver condition. This is not a quick fix; however, it will take time to see positive results from your lifestyle changes, but they will come.

HOW TO SUCCESSFULLY COMBAT A FATTY LIVER

FATTY LIVER IS a special condition characterized by the build-up of fat on the underlying tissues of the liver, which becomes a health concern and risk. This build-up of fat occurs gradually but seems to proceed rather quickly in obese individuals or people with abnormal weight. In most cases, the build-up is unnoticeable and without symptoms, but later the manifestation of the condition becomes evident after symptoms start emerging. This condition can be managed effectively if an early diagnosis is made and treatment follows immediately.

Reverse your fatty liver and boost your liver function with proper dieting.

Just like other diet-related health problems, this condition can be combated effectively by adopting a combination of foods that boost liver function while at the same time mitigating the effects of the fat build-up. The secret to overcoming this disease is to know which foods to eat and which ones to avoid, and their correct proportions. The good news is that just like obesity, this can be overcome.

The first thing you should do when combating your fatty liver is to cut down on your fat consumption. You will find that if you are obese, then the chances are that you have considerable fat deposits on tissues and organs, including the liver. In short, individuals with abnormal weight are more prevalent to this condition, even if the symptoms are not yet evident.

It's not enough to cut down on the consumption of fatty foods in your quest to overcome this liver condition. The reason is that you may suffer the effects of immediate withdrawal, such as hunger. Well, to overcome this challenge, you should embrace a fat-free wholesome diet that will supply the desired calories, keep your stomach full, boost your overall health, and allow the liver to function optimally. Fresh organic vegetables, fruits, and wholemeal bread can help you reduce fat buildup and keep you healthy.

Adopt a more liver-friendly diet to combat your fatty liver

There are specific organic foods that you should embrace wholly in your diet if you want to mitigate the effects of fat build-up and liver deterioration or fatty liver disease. Although you may find these foods unpalatable at first, you will find their effects revitalizing once you get used to them. Fresh organic vegetables and fruits, whole-grains supply nutrients and ensure the proper functioning of the liver. You should adopt a diet that is more liver-friendly to keep it in good shape.

You should avoid taking or stop taking alcohol if you stand a high risk of developing a liver condition. Alcohol can degenerate the condition of your liver and make treatment very difficult. This is true, especially if you are diagnosed with liver cirrhosis caused by excessive alcohol consumption. If you have been drinking and are also overweight, you should quit drinking altogether.

In case of severe liver damage, you are advised to go for extensive treatment to prevent the situation or condition of your liver from worsening. Your physician should be in a position to determine the kind of medication you need, depending on the stage of the condition. It may be difficult to reverse the effects of later stages of this liver disease, but it is possible to stop further liver damage.

Exercise coupled with a proper diet will reverse your fatty liver.

If the fatty liver is due to obesity, you have to adopt an exercise program in conjunction with your fatty liver diet to eliminate fat buildup. Regular workouts will help your body burn more calories and ensure only the necessary amount of calories is stored in your body. If you adopt the routine with persistence, then the deposition of fat will gradually reduce until your fatty liver condition is overcome by breaking down stored fat.

Fatty Liver - Natural Cures for Fatty Liver

When looking for a natural cure for fatty liver, you need to see how to cleanse the liver of fat, regenerate damaged liver cells and protect the liver from further damage.

These are some very powerful herbs and supplements considered when looking for natural cures for fatty liver.

- *Milk Thistle*

Milk thistle is a well-known natural remedy for the treatment of liver disorders. The active ingredient found in the seeds is the phytochemical silymarin. Silymarin is a flavonoid that promotes the regeneration of damaged liver cells and improves liver function.

Silymarin has been shown in clinical research studies to help regenerate liver cells. Many, but not all, clinical studies have proven measurable improvement in liver function tests when silymarin is given to people with alcohol-induced liver damage. Silymarin is a derivative from the milk thistle plant with few adverse reactions and has been used for centuries to treat liver ailments.

In France, Germany, Hungary, and Greece, various formulations of milk thistle are used for a wide variety of liver ailments. In Europe, milk thistle is currently used as a protective and regenerative agent for liver damage due to hepatitis, cirrhosis of the liver, alcohol, drugs, and environmental toxins. These uses are becoming ever more popular in the United States due to the great interest in natural cures.

- *Omega-3 Fatty Acids*

Omega-3 fatty acids are found naturally in flax seeds, plant oils like flaxseed and canola oils, fish oils, and cold-water fish like salmon. Omega-3 fatty acids are known to have excellent liver health benefits, improve insulin activity, and assist many people who suffer from fatty liver disease. Moreover, Omega-3 fatty acids decrease inflammation and pain among those suffering from a fatty liver condition.

- *Flax Seeds*

Flax seeds are high in Omega-3 fatty acids and are great natural food sources to protect the liver, reduce inflammation and cure fatty liver. Ground flax seeds can be incorporated into almost any recipe. If you love your oatmeal, start adding ground flax! It will give your oatmeal a nutty, richer flavor while increasing your fiber and Omega-3 intake.

Flaxseed oil contains significant amounts of Omega-3 fatty acids as well as high-grade micronutrients and vitamins. Flaxseed oil is also used to help lower high levels of cholesterol and balance metabolism, especially in women. Flaxseed oil is especially tasty on a green salad.

- *Vitamin E*

Vitamin E is especially beneficial for the liver because it protects against free radicals during the natural detox process. It is an antioxidant, meaning it protects against free radical damage. Vitamin E is also beneficial for the immune system and can help prevent fibrosis and cirrhosis of the liver, common complications of long-term fatty liver.

These are some very powerful things to consider when choosing a natural cure for fatty liver. You can regain your health by supplementing your diet with these natural foods. Each one is excellent for cleansing, restoring, and rejuvenating the liver.

The simple truth is, your liver has a remarkable power to heal. If you are suffering from fatty liver, it is especially important to start caring for your liver now--before the fatty buildup causes more damage to your liver.

Diets For People With Fatty Liver - 4 Keys To Removing Excess Fat From Your Liver

The best diet for reducing a fatty liver promotes overall health and not just healthy liver function. But before the proper diet can be determined, it's important first to understand what a fatty liver is.

HEALTH AND WELLNESS LIFE

Fatty liver (also known as fatty liver disease or FLD) refers to an over-abundance of triglyceride fats in the liver. These fats accumulate via steatosis and take up space in and around hepatocytes (liver cells). This causes the liver to become larger and heavier.

The condition progresses through four stages that range from simple fatty liver (steatosis) to fatty liver coupled with inflammation (steatohepatitis). It can also be caused by alcohol consumption (AFL) or without alcohol (NAFLD).

Steatosis itself is asymptomatic and benign, but later stages of the disease can be life-threatening as they can lead to cirrhosis and liver cancer. Due to a rise in obesity in the United States, fatty liver disease has become the most common cause for liver tests over the last decade.

Because the disease is largely asymptomatic, especially in its earliest stages, many people have no idea they have the affliction until it has already progressed. Performing a liver biopsy is the only method for getting a definitive diagnosis.

The good news is science has proven liver fat can be reduced, and the condition can be improved through a proper diet. A good diet for reducing a fatty liver will follow some key principles. **The following can put you on the right path.**

- *Foods High In Fiber And Rich In Complex Carbohydrates*

A healthy liver diet should comprise 60-70% complex carbohydrates (think pasta and brown rice) and foods rich in fiber. Fiber aids in the digestion process, which can help burn and remove excess fat. Simple carbohydrates like those found in most sweets should be avoided.

- *Control The Calories*

A good diet to reduce fat in the liver will be highly nutritional, balanced and will control caloric intake. Reducing calories will help you lose weight which will reduce stress on your liver. Shoot for between 1200 and 1500 calories per day.

- *Reduce The Fat*

FLD is often associated with obesity, so reducing your overall fat intake can help you lose weight and keep excess fat from ending up in your liver. Try to keep the fat content to less than 30% of your overall caloric intake.

- *Fruits And Vegetables For Vitamins And Minerals*

Vitamins and minerals are also extremely important for the liver. The best sources for these come from greens and leaves, and citrus fruits high in vitamin C. Vegetables such as beans can also be an excellent alternative source of protein.

Fatty Liver Disease Diet Tips - How To Reduce Liver Fat By Watching What You Eat

A good fatty liver disease diet can be implemented to stop and/or reverse excessive fat in the liver without keeping you from enjoying many of the foods you love. Like a healthy diet for the average person, moderation and balance are the keys.

Although you will need to find more healthy alternatives for some of the things you eat and keep a closer eye on your food consumption, you'll still find many delicious liver-friendly recipes to satisfy your taste buds.

Fatty liver disease (FLD) generally falls into one of two categories based on its cause. When alcohol consumption is the main culprit of excess fat in the liver, the disease is classified as alcoholic fatty liver (AFL). Suppose other factors such as a high-fat diet, obesity, diabetes millets, metabolic disorders, hyperlipidemia, or hypertension are the culprit. In that case, the disease is classified as non-alcoholic fatty liver disease (NAFLD).

AFL is generally considered easier to treat because of its singular cause. Often asymptomatic and benign in early stages, both types can become fatal in the form of cirrhosis, liver cancer, hepatocellular carcinoma, and total liver failure if left unchecked.

However, when caught early, simple changes in diet and exercise aimed at losing weight are often needed to slow or even reverse the condition. Fat reduction and weight loss must be made gradually to keep the body from going into an internal state similar to starvation.

When this happens, the body makes up for the lost fat by rapidly producing fatty acids, which worsen fatty liver. This is why drastic measures of weight loss such as gastric bypass surgery are not often recommended for FLD patients.

A diet plan for fatty liver should reduce fat consumption to no more than 20-30% of the daily caloric intake. This means if you're eating a 1500 calorie diet, then no more than 450 of those calories should come from fats, especially saturated fats. Replace high-fat foods with high-fiber foods.

The main energy source for FLD patients should come from complex carbohydrates such as those found in brown rice and pasta. These should make up approximately 60-70% of the overall diet. In our example above, this means 900-1050 of the 1500 calorie diet should come from complex carbohydrates.

Avoid foods containing only simple carbohydrates. These are found in things like candy and other sweets. Simple carbohydrates break down quickly and are used too fast by the body. Once these carbohydrates are used, the body starts feeling starved, and fatty acid production occurs in the liver. As we mentioned earlier, this is an undesirable condition for fatty liver disease patients.

FATTY LIVER DISEASE IS A TICKING TIME BOMB: GET YOURSELF EXAMINED TODAY

FATTY LIVER DISEASE is often ignored for its slow evolution process. Since the ailment is time-dependent, a patient misunderstands the initial curveballs typically that this disease throws out. To make matters more complicated, Fatty Liver problems aren't strongly tied to alcoholics.

IN BIOLOGICAL TERMS, LIVER DISEASE IS REFERRED TO AS Alcoholic Liver Disease. By default, every healthy human being has a thin film of fat molecules covering the muscle area. If the imbiber takes too many carbs and drinks many heavy beverages on the alcohol, the amount of fat inside the liver increases exponentially.

THIS INCREASED AMOUNT OF FATTY TISSUES CAN RESULT IN A variation of liver-related problems. However, it was mentioned earlier that the problem isn't strongly reliant on alcohol intake. Henceforth, any obese person could be the next victim of this vile disease.

· · ·

Due to overgrowing obesity levels, 35% of individuals in America are prone to liver diseases. **The initial symptoms of this disease can be dished out as:**

- Consistent level of discomfort and fatigue
- Dizziness and "weird gut" feeling in the upper abdominal cavity

In addition to the above symptoms, a normal version (non-alcoholic) of fatty liver is regarded as Steatosis. Regardless of your drinking antics, patients with Steatosis based profile can also develop **the following features under the non-alcoholic fatty liver category:**

- Rashes on skin with the itchy feeling
- Vomit normally consists of blood strings
- Skin becomes hypersensitive to bruises
- Memory loss
- Body loses muscle retention process. Palms get mottled, and skin develops a yellowish color

An advanced stage of fatty liver disease is called fibrosis. It normally occurs when the liver delves into the Non-Alcoholic Hepatitis stage, which further develops scar tissues inside the liver. A consistency in fibrosis condition can lead to severe and often irreversible damage to the liver. **The abdominal ailment spreads over the following series of changes:**

- Initial weight loss problems give vent to the first stage of fatty liver disease
- With a Body Mass Index of 25.0+, the patient advances to the next level, which is T-2 Diabetes
- At this point, the affected body becomes resistant to insulin treatment
- Liver goes into fibrosis stage and increases blood pressure levels

Cure:

There is no permanent short-termed cure for this disease. The patient has to be exposed to a series of drugs over a scheduled interval of various months. After carrying out several tests that are spread over Ultrasound, blood tests, CAT, and CT scans, doctors issue their prescription.

If your fatty liver disease were strictly a result of alcohol inhibition, you'd be advised to hold up on alcohol intake immediately. Mild cases are normally treated through prevention and medicine-based prescriptions. Patients are always instructed to follow a decent diet and exercise regimen, which would result in rapid weight loss.

. . .

What To Eat To Improve A Fatty Liver - Eat This, Don't Eat That, What Every FLD Patient Should Know.

If you're wondering what to eat to improve a fatty liver, then take just a few moments to read to the end of this article. Here are some of the foods you should and should not eat to reduce fat in your liver:

A fatty liver refers to having too much fat (specifical triglycerides) accumulated in your liver. So what exactly is "too much" fat? Generally speaking, a liver is considered "fatty" when fat makes up between 5-10% or more of the liver by weight. Fat builds up in and around the spaces of hepatocytes (liver cells), causing the liver to enlarge and grow heavier.

In the early stages of FLD, often referred to as simple steatosis, the condition is often benign and asymptomatic. Many patients don't even know they have FLD. It is often found when doing blood work or other tests for entirely different reasons. The only way to definitively diagnose the condition is through a liver biopsy, but factors such as elevated liver enzymes often clue physicians into the problem.

A diet plan for fatty liver is most often centered around balance, moderation, regulation, and reducing fat intake to less than 30% of the total daily calories. In other words, if you're eating a 1200 calorie diet, then fat calories should make up no more than 360 of those calories. This is equivalent to about 40 grams per day.

Since the fatty liver is often associated with obesity, losing weight can significantly impact liver function and liver health.

So that brings us to the question of what you should and should not eat. Complex carbohydrates should make up the bulk of your energy source. These can be found in things like whole grains, brown rice, and pasta. The simple carbohydrates found in sweets should be avoided.

Diets for fatty liver patients are also generally high in fiber and include an abundance of fruits and vegetables. Fats, particularly saturated fats, should be carefully monitored. Protein can be obtained from vegetables or leaner white meats such as chicken or turkey instead of beef or pork. Here is a brief rundown of some of the things you should and should not eat if you want to reduce fat in your liver.

Foods You Should Avoid And/Or Carefully Monitor

- White bread and white rice
- High-fat butter
- Sweets containing simple carbohydrates (candy, doughnuts, etc.)
- High-fat foods (pizza, ribs, pot pies, etc.)
- Eggs and other high cholesterol foods
- Sugary and/or carbonated drinks such as soda
- Fast foods and/or processed meats such as hot dogs
- Fried foods
- Alcohol (particularly if you have alcoholic fatty liver (AFL))

- Salad dressing and other high-fat condiments (look for low-fat or non-fat alternatives)
- Red meats (beef, pork)

Foods To Eat To Improve A Fatty Liver

- Vegetables (greens, leaves, legumes, tomatoes, and especially broccoli)
- Fruits rich in vitamin E and vitamin C (oranges, papaya, kiwi, mango)
- Beans (these are a great alternative source of protein)
- Whole-grain bread
- Milk in moderation (whole substitute milk or 2% milk with either skims milk or 1% milk)
- Brown rice and pasta
- Lean white meats (chicken, turkey, tuna)

Fatty Liver Diet - How to Treat Fatty Liver Disease

To treat, reverse, and cure a fatty liver, patients must understand that a lifestyle change is necessary for their eating habits and exercise routines. Failure to adopt a healthier living plan can worsen the disease to cirrhosis, liver failure, and death, as there are no surgeries or medications proven to cure it. Patients that implement a specific fatty liver diet plan and incorporate light exercise will eliminate Fatty Liver Disease.

. . .

Fatty Liver Diet

The diet plan has some particular guidelines to follow that begin to work immediately to slow the progression of the disease. While changing your diet can be somewhat uncomfortable, the best suggestion is to find the meals and recipes you like that fall under the specific diet requirements. **The food intake should be considered using these guidelines:**

- Foods high in protein
- Heavy consumption of fruits and vegetables
- Food that is high in fiber
- Low-cholesterol foods
- Low-calorie foods

Making subtle and drastic changes in your daily meal plans, reading more labels on food containers, and understanding the diet requirements will keep you on track in reversing the disease. **Consider removing these aspects from your daily diet regimen:**

- Carbonated drinks
- Fried food, fast food
- White bread, white rice
- Concentrated sugars
- Fat-rich, high-cholesterol foods
- High-glycerin food
- Butter, whole milk

Exercising to Treat a Fatty Liver

Exercising is just as important as dieting when treating the disease; however, it should be light and not too rigorous. Taking it slow and performing basic exercises daily will keep you focused and balance your body's natural healing process to eliminate the disease.

Start by choosing a form of exercise you enjoy doing that you look forward to in your spare time. For example, you could join a bowling league, play racquetball, softball, etc. The trick to prolonging healthy exercise in your life is truly enjoying it and not just running out and joining a health club or gym unless you enjoy doing it. Most people find discouragement and lose interest quickly with exercise routines and activities that are not fun or just too demanding.

Knowledge, Balance, Commitment

Start your fatty liver diet the right way: Plan out your meals daily and read more labels on your buy items. Make that commitment for exercising, and track your progress with your doctor. Treating a fatty liver does not have to be scary or even hard to do, but it should be treated with a sense of pleasure to help you keep the commitment.

Natural Remedies for Fatty Liver Disease

. . .

HEALTH AND WELLNESS LIFE

If you have NAFLD, keep in mind that not all diets and supplements are healthy for your liver. It's important to discuss any alternative treatments with your healthcare provider before trying them.

- *Lose excess weight.*

The American Association for the Study of Liver Diseases (AASLD) identifies weight loss as a critical part of improving NAFLD progression and symptoms.

The guide recommends that people with NAFLD lose between 3 and 5 percent of their body weight to reduce fat buildup in the liver. It also states that losing between 7 and 10 percent of body weight can improve other symptoms of NAFLD, such as inflammation, fibrosis, and scarring.

The best way to lose weight and maintain it is to take small steps toward your goal over time. Fasting and extreme diets are often unsustainable, and they can be hard on your liver.

Before beginning any weight loss program, it's important to speak with your healthcare provider to see if it's right for you. A dietitian can develop an eating plan to help you reach your weight loss goals and make nutritious food choices.

- *Try the Mediterranean diet.*

RESEARCH SUGGESTS THAT THE MEDITERRANEAN DIET MAY HELP TO reduce liver fat, even without weight loss.

THE MEDITERRANEAN DIET ALSO HELPS TREAT CONDITIONS COMMONLY associated with NAFLD, including high cholesterol, high blood pressure, and type 2 diabetes. This eating plan focuses on various plant-based foods, including fresh fruits and vegetables and legumes, along with healthy fats. **Here's a brief overview of foods to focus on:**

- Fruits and vegetables. Aim to eat variously: Try berries, apples, oranges, bananas, dates, figs, melons, leafy greens, broccoli, peppers, sweet potatoes, carrots, squash, cucumbers, eggplant, and tomatoes.
- Legumes. Try to include beans, peas, lentils, pulses, and chickpeas in your diet.
- Healthy fats. Use healthy oils, such as extra virgin olive oil. Nuts, seeds, avocados, and olives also contain a high concentration of healthy fats.
- Fish and lean meats. Opt for fish twice per week. Eggs and lean poultry, like skinless chicken and turkey, are fine in moderation.
- Whole grains. Consume unprocessed grains and cereals, such as whole-wheat bread, brown rice, whole oats, couscous, whole-wheat pasta, or quinoa.

- *Drink coffee.*

According to research, coffee offers several protective benefits for the liver. In particular, it stimulates the production of liver enzymes believed to fight inflammation.

The same research reported that among people with NAFLD, regular coffee consumption reduces overall liver damage.

Aim to drink two to three cups of coffee per day to lower the risk of liver disease. Black coffee is the best option, as it doesn't contain any added fat or sugar.

- *Get active.*

According to research, NAFLD is often associated with a sedentary lifestyle. Also, inactivity is known to contribute to other conditions associated with NAFLD, including heart disease, type 2 diabetes, and obesity.

It's important to stay active when you have NAFLD. According to a study, a good goal to shoot for is at least 150 minutes of moderate-intensity exercise per week.

That's around 30 minutes, 5 days per week. You don't necessarily have to play a sport or even go to the gym to get enough exercise. You can take a brisk 30-minute walk, 5 days a week.

. . .

Or, if you're pressed for time, you can even break it down into two brisk 15-minute walks, twice a day, 5 days a week.

To start exercising, try integrating moderate physical activity into your daily routine. Walk to the grocery store, walk the dog, play with your kids, or take the stairs instead of the elevator whenever you can.

The guidelines also recommend reducing the amount of time you spend sitting during the day.

- *Avoid foods with added sugars.*

Dietary sugars such as fructose and sucrose have been linked to the development of NAFLD. Research describes how these sugars contribute to fat buildup in the liver.

Major culprits include store-bought and commercially processed foods, **such as:**

- baked goods, like cakes, cookies, doughnuts, pastries, and pies
- candy
- ice cream
- sugary cereals
- soft drinks
- sports drinks

- energy drinks
- sweetened dairy products, like flavored yogurts

To identify whether a packaged food contains added sugar, read the ingredients list on the product packaging. Words that end in "ose," including sucrose, fructose, and maltose, are sugars. **Other sugars commonly added to food products include:**

- cane sugar
- high-fructose corn syrup
- corn sweetener
- fruit juice concentrate
- honey
- molasses
- syrup

Another way to tell how much sugar is in a food item is to read the nutrition facts label and look at the number of grams of sugar serving that item — the lower, the better.

- *Target high cholesterol.*

According to research, NAFLD makes it harder for your body to manage cholesterol on its own. This can worsen NAFLD and increase your risk of heart disease.

. . .

Try to limit your intake of certain types of fats to help control your cholesterol and treat NAFLD. **Fats to avoid include:**

- Saturated fats. These are found in meats and full-fat dairy products.
- Trans fats. Trans fats are often found in processed baked goods, crackers, and fried foods.

Many of the lifestyle changes listed above — including losing weight, staying active, and adopting a Mediterranean diet — can also help you manage your cholesterol. Your doctor might also prescribe medication for high cholesterol.

- *Try an omega-3 supplement.*

Some types of fats can be beneficial to your health. Omega-3 fatty acids are polyunsaturated fats found in foods such as oily fish and some nuts and seeds. They're known to have benefits for heart health and are recommended for people with NAFLD.

A study suggests that taking an omega-3 supplement can reduce liver fat and improve cholesterol levels.

In the review, daily omega-3 doses ranged from 830 to 9,000 milligrams. Talk to your doctor about how much you should take.

- *Avoid known liver irritants.*

CERTAIN SUBSTANCES CAN PUT EXCESS STRESS ON YOUR LIVER. SOME of these substances include alcohol, over-the-counter medications, and some vitamins and supplements.

ACCORDING TO RESEARCH, IT'S BEST TO AVOID ALCOHOL altogether if you have NAFLD. While moderate alcohol consumption may benefit healthy people, it isn't clear if those benefits also apply to people with NAFLD.

ALSO, SPEAK TO A DOCTOR OR PHARMACIST BEFORE TAKING ANY OVER-the-counter medication, vitamins, or supplements, as these can affect your liver.

- *Ask your doctor about vitamin E supplements.*

VITAMIN E IS AN ANTIOXIDANT THAT MAY REDUCE INFLAMMATION caused by NAFLD. According to a study, more research is needed to understand who can benefit from this treatment.

IN A STUDY, THE AASLD RECOMMENDS A DAILY DOSE OF 800 international units of vitamin E per day for people with NAFLD. They don't have diabetes and have confirmed nonalcoholic steatohepatitis (NASH), an advanced form of NAFLD.

THERE ARE RISKS ASSOCIATED WITH THIS TREATMENT. TALK TO YOUR doctor to determine if vitamin E is right for you and whether it could help with your NAFLD.

- *Try herbs and supplements.*

A study identified herbs, supplements, and spices that have been used as alternative treatments for NAFLD. Compounds shown to affect liver health positively include turmeric, milk thistle, resveratrol, and green tea.

Remember that these aren't approved medical treatments for NAFLD, and they may have side effects. It's important to talk to your doctor before taking any herbs and supplements for NAFLD.

Medical Treatments

There are currently no approved medical treatments for NAFLD, though there are some in development.

One such treatment is pioglitazone, a medication typically prescribed for type 2 diabetes. The AASLD suggests that pioglitazone may help improve liver health in people with and without type 2 diabetes.

More research needs to be done to understand the long-term safety and effectiveness of this treatment. As a result, this medication is only recommended for people with confirmed NASH.

HEALTH AND WELLNESS LIFE

. . .

5 Fat Reducing Remedies For Your Liver

Various treatments and remedies continue to be tested, and some are showing positive results. Until science proves otherwise, fatty liver disease (FLD) will continue to be a rather asymptomatic disease in its early stages that can turn lethal in the form of cirrhosis, liver cancer, and liver failure if not kept in check.

Here are 5 fat-reducing remedies commonly used to treat excess fat in the liver:

- *Epsom Salts*

Epsom salts are sometimes recommended as a type of "liver flush" to remove fats and toxins from liver tissues. Epsom salts work by solidifying cholesterol into small stones that are then excreted. This treatment can be done at home, although some patients experience discomfort during excretion and occasionally feel sick afterward.

- *Milk Thistle*

Milk thistle is a herb containing silymarin which is a liver-friendly compound with excellent antioxidant properties. Milk thistle treatment aims to protect the liver from damage and toxins and assist in regenerating damaged hepatocytes (liver cells). It keeps the liver healthy so the liver can better deal with conditions like fatty liver and cirrhosis.

- *Vitamin E and Vitamin C*

THE THIRD LIVER REMEDY IS VITAMIN E AND VITAMIN C SUPPLEMENTS. Much like silymarin in milk thistle, these serve as antioxidants to protect the liver from damage and deterioration.

- *Prescription Drugs*

A WIDE VARIETY OF DRUGS HAVE BEEN PRESCRIBED AS WAYS TO treat fatty liver. They generally aim at combating problems resulting from a damaged liver. **These include drugs like:**

- Orlistat
- Metformin
- Rosiglitazone
- Pioglitazone
- Gemfibrozil
- Atorvastatin
- Pravastatin

- *Diet And Exercise*

The most common and widely accepted treatment for reducing fat in the liver is proper diet and exercise. This remedy also still has the most positive results for improving and sometimes even reversing the condition.

Controlling excess fat in the liver through this method focuses on removing fatty foods from the diet and following an exercise program for gradual weight reduction. This method improves overall health and not just the health of your liver.

How To Have A Healthy Liver

The liver is the key organ for detoxification. If toxins are allowed to build up in the body, we might suffer from fatigue, bad breath, weight gain, cellulite, headaches, leaky gut, acne, and a general lack of energy and wellness. Read on for simple but super effective ways to improve your liver function and take a giant leap towards great health and wellbeing.

The following health tips will help optimize your liver function, which will clear your toxins body:

- **Maintain a healthy weight.** If you're obese or even somewhat overweight, you're in danger of having a fatty liver that can lead to non-alcoholic fatty liver disease (NAFLD), one of the fastest-growing forms of liver disease. Weight loss can play an important part in helping to reduce liver fat.

- **Eat a balanced diet.** Avoid high calorie-meals, saturated fat, refined carbohydrates (such as white bread, white rice, and regular pasta), and sugars. Don't eat raw or undercooked shellfish. For a well-adjusted diet, eat fiber, which you can obtain from fresh fruits, vegetables, whole-grain bread, rice, and cereals. Also, eat meat (but limit the amount of red meat), dairy (low-fat milk and small amounts of cheese), and fats (the "good" fats that are monounsaturated and polyunsaturated such as vegetable oils, nuts, seeds, and fish). Hydration is essential, so drink a lot of water.

- **Exercise regularly.** When you exercise consistently, it helps to burn triglycerides for fuel and can also reduce liver fat.

- **Avoid toxins.** Toxins can injure liver cells. Limit direct contact with toxins from cleaning and aerosol products, insecticides, chemicals, and additives. When you do use aerosols, make sure the room is ventilated and wear a mask. Don't smoke.

- **Use alcohol responsibly.** Alcoholic beverages can create many health problems. They can damage or destroy liver cells and scar your liver. Talk to your doctor about what amount of alcohol is right for you. You may be advised to drink alcohol only in moderation or to quit completely.

- **Avoid the use of illegal drugs.** In 2016, nearly 24 million Americans aged 12 or older were current illicit drug users, meaning they had used an illegal drug during the month before the survey interview. This estimate represents 9.2 percent of the population aged 12 or older. Illicit drugs include marijuana/hashish, cocaine (including crack), heroin, hallucinogens, inhalants, or prescription-type psychotherapeutics (pain relievers, tranquilizers, stimulants, and sedatives) used non-medically.

- **Avoid contaminated needles.** Of course, dirty needles aren't only associated with intravenous drug use. You should follow up with a medical practitioner and seek testing following any skin penetration involving sharp instruments or needles. Unsafe injection practices, though rare, may occur in a hospital setting and would need immediate follow-up. Also, use only clean needles for tattoos and body piercings.

- **Get medical care if you're exposed to blood.** If, for any reason, you come into contact with someone else's blood, immediately follow up with your doctor. If you're very concerned, go to your nearest hospital's emergency room.

- **Don't share personal hygiene items.** For example, razors, toothbrushes, and nail clippers can carry microscopic levels of blood or other body fluids that may be contaminated.

- **Practice safe sex.** Unprotected sex or sex with multiple partners increases your risk of hepatitis B and hepatitis C.

- **Wash your hands.** Use soap and warm water immediately after using the bathroom, when you have changed a diaper, and before preparing or eating food.

- **Follow directions on all medications.** When medicines are taken incorrectly by taking too much, the wrong type, or mixing medicines, your liver can be harmed. Never mix alcohol with other drugs and medications even if they're not taken at the same time. Tell your doctor about any over-the-counter medicines, supplements, and natural or herbal remedies that you use.

- **Get vaccinated.** There are vaccines for hepatitis A and hepatitis B. Unfortunately, there's no vaccine against the hepatitis C virus.

TREAT YOUR LIVER WELL, AND YOU ARE TREATING YOUR ENTIRE BODY well. A healthy liver will process the toxins so they will leave your body without causing harm.

CONCLUSION

People with fatty liver disease showed a markedly higher risk of developing liver-related death than the general population. The AFLD group had higher liver-related mortality and had a worse survival than the NAFLD group. People with more severe fibrosis at baseline showed a worse survival than patients with none or mild fibrosis.

Nonalcoholic fatty liver disease affects 20–30% of adult populations in developed countries. The build-up of fat in the liver is harmless at first, but it can lead to nonalcoholic steatohepatitis (inflammation and liver damage).

Fatty liver disease is so intimately associated with type 2 diabetes, obesity, hyperlipidemia, metabolic syndrome, and heart disease caused by the same factors. These factors are an unhealthy lifestyle, genetics, and gut health issues (obesity and inflammation-causing microbiome).

CONCLUSION

Although genetics can't be changed, almost everyone can prevent and reverse fatty liver disease with the right diet and exercise program. Research suggests that the right diet is a low carbohydrate and high fiber diet. The perfect example of this is the ketogenic diet. This diet maintains a healthy gut microbiome and limits fructose and carbohydrate (the two dietary components that cause fat to build up in the liver), making it the ideal fatty liver diet.

Many different forms of activity, from walking to lifting weights, can help reverse fatty liver disease when it comes to exercise. Do some form of activity every day for best results.

Combining the ketogenic diet plan and exercise makes a great treatment for fatty liver disease, but they aren't the only important things that can help reverse the disease. Limiting alcohol intake, eating low-carbohydrate vegetables like spinach and kale, taking liver healing supplements like spirulina and milk thistle, and including liver healing foods in your diet are essential in reversing fatty liver disease as well.

When you put it all together, **here is an overly simplified version of the best fatty liver diet and lifestyle plan:**

- Restrict carbohydrates
- Eat low-carbohydrate vegetables with every meal
- Exercise every day
- Take scientifically-proven liver healing supplements like spirulina, betaine, and milk thistle
- Include liver healing foods in your diet like avocado, nuts, oily fish, olive oil, and unsweetened coffee
- Limit alcohol intake

CONCLUSION

Lifestyle and dietary changes are currently the most effective treatment options for NAFLD. Losing weight, being physically active, cutting back on sugar, eating a healthier diet, and drinking coffee are some of the ways that may help improve symptoms associated with NALFD.

If you have this condition, be sure to work closely with your doctor to develop a personalized treatment plan that's right for you.

Lightning Source UK Ltd.
Milton Keynes UK
UKHW051238100422
401245UK00014B/2480